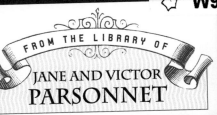

THE
JEWISH
DOCTOR

THE JEWISH DOCTOR

A Narrative History

Michael Nevins

JASON ARONSON INC.
Northvale, New Jersey
London

The author gratefully acknowledges permission to quote from the following sources:

The Last Angry Man, by Gerald Green. Copyright 1956 Gerald Green; copyright © 1984. Reprinted with permission of Scribner, an imprint of Simon & Schuster.

"I Remember: Nostalgic Memories of Half a Century in New York," by Israel Augenblick, M.D. Copyright © 1965 Jeffrey A. Marx. Used by permission of the American Jewish Archives, Cincinnati, Ohio, and Jeffrey A. Marx.

This book was set in 12 pt. Garamond.

Library of Congress Cataloging-in-Publication Data

Nevins, Michael A.
    The Jewish doctor : a narrative history / Michael Nevins.
        p.   cm.
    Includes bibliographical references and index.
    ISBN 1-56821-533-9 (alk. paper)
    1. Jewish physicians—History.   2. Jews—Medicine—History.
    I. Title.
    R694.N48   1996
    610.69'52'089924—dc20   95-46149

Manufactured in the United States of America. Jason Aronson Inc. offers books and cassettes. For information and catalog write to Jason Aronson Inc., 230 Livingston Street, Northvale, New Jersey 07647.

To
my wonderful family

Contents

vii

Acknowledgments

The materials included in this collection were found with the assistance of many librarians in institutions as small as the River Vale, New Jersey, Public Library and the libraries of Temple Emanuel of the Pascack Valley and Pascack Valley Hospital, Westwood, New Jersey, and as grand as the Jewish Theological Seminary in New York and the American Jewish Archives in Cincinnati, Ohio. I am indebted to them all. At various times a number of individuals provided helpful information, including Lisa Epstein, Dr. Saul Jarcho, Stanley Batkin, Dr. Leon Sokoloff, Al Beckman, and Dr. Aaron Feingold. In particular, I'd like to thank David Cowen and my son Rabbi Daniel Nevins for their excellent manuscript review and good advice.

Introduction

A frequently quoted story attributed to a sixteenth-century observer relates that when the French king, King Francis I, suffered from a lingering illness, he sent a courier to Spain to ask the Holy Roman Emperor Charles V to send his most skilled Jewish physician. When the doctor arrived, the king jokingly asked if he were not yet tired of waiting for the Messiah. The doctor, who was a *converso* or "New Christian," pointed out that he no longer was a Jew, having converted to "the only true faith." Indignantly, the king dismissed him and sent to Constantinople for a *real* Jewish physician. The legitimate Jewish doctor reportedly found it necessary to prescribe nothing other than ass's milk.[1] Whether the story is true or apocryphal, it illustrates that throughout history there was a prevailing sense that there was something special and distinguishing about Jewish doctors.

Among gentiles, Jewish doctors either were admired or reviled, sometimes simultaneously. Their fortunes varied according to the times, and since they frequently had to combat ignorance and intolerance, until this century they were often more innovative in their survival techniques than in their original contributions to medical progress. During the ninth through eleventh centuries, under the relatively congenial Arabic hegemony in the Middle East and Spain, Jewish doctors were esteemed translators and transmitters of classical Greek medicine. In medieval and Renaissance Europe, even as laws were passed restricting their capacity to practice, Jewish court physicians were sought after by monarchs and popes who valued their services. After the French Revolution and the Enlightenment, when Jews increasingly were granted civil rights and educational opportunities, they used the medical profession as a means of upward social mobility or of escape to physical and intellectual freedom.

In 1914 Sir William Osler said, "In the medical profession the Jews had a long and honorable record, and among no people is all that is best in our science and art more warmly appreciated."[2] Rudolf Virchow, speaking in 1894, attributed Jewish medical success to "a hereditary talent." However, whether or not Jews truly have a unique aptitude for medicine is arguable. To be sure, the Bible and the Talmud are replete with medical advice, talmudic discourse promotes a kind of intense analysis that is well suited to science, and the traditional Jewish zest for learning has served Jews particularly well in medical studies.

If ability and opportunism were important determinants of Jewish affinity for medical practice, for many individuals the price of bursting out of the ghettos was that traditional customs and values either were jettisoned or altogether rejected. The erudite rabbi physician-scholars of medieval times became supplanted by aculturated secular scientists, and it appears as if the intellectual passion that once was expended on religious study became transferred to worldly affairs.

Contributions by Jewish scientists in this century often are taken for granted, but they have been exceptional. The most obvious evidence is the vastly disproportionate number of Jewish Nobel Prize winners—nearly one-quarter of all recipients of the prize for medicine and physiology (34 of 150 from 1901 to 1990)—from a group that comprises only a fraction of 1 percent of the world's population.[3] Jewish physicians helped to make German medicine preeminent during the late nineteenth and early twentieth centuries, and certainly they were major contributors to the development of science in the United States in the modern era.

Still, few knowledgeable people today can name even a single Jewish physician who lived before this century other than Maimonides or Freud. My purpose in these essays will be to familiarize a general audience with the lives and practices of certain Jewish physicians in the context of their times. Conventional medical history emphasizes the biographies of famous doctors, but I will also address what has been called "the sociology of medicine." Historian Henry Sigerist considered medicine not so much a natural as a social science and insisted that equal attention should be paid to doctor's relationships with their patients and their communities as to their individual exploits or to who discovered something first.[4] It has also been said, "If social history is history with the politics left out, the social history of medicine is medical history with the public interest put in."[5]

The literature of Jewish medical history is extensive. However, standard reference texts by venerable scholars such as Moritz Steinschneider, Julius Preuss,

Solomon Kagen, and Harry Friedenwald were published fifty to one hundred years or more ago. In our own time books and articles, notably by Fred Rosner, have focused on biblical and talmudic medicine and the writings of Maimonides. The genre also includes sporadic articles that have appeared generally in rather obscure specialty journals. I have borrowed liberally from all of these sources, and the present contribution, in effect, is an introductory sampler both of the older and of the more recent material. As explained before, it differs from conventional works in that it includes descriptions of folk practices that rarely are mentioned in discussions of mainstream medicine.

This eclectic collection is not intended to provide a comprehensive review of every aspect of Jewish medical history. By focusing on medical practitioners and their work, many other important subjects were omitted, such as the contribution of Jewish institutions and organizations, bioethics and medical research, as well as detailed discussion of the Holocaust and modern Israel. All of these certainly are worthy of review in a more definitive, larger work. My selection method was merely to choose material that appealed to me as being fresh, interesting, or relevant to contemporary issues. No doubt, others would have chosen differently.

The chapters appear roughly in chronological order, and my intent has been to create the effect of a medical montage. The information-gathering process afforded me a vicarious chance to experience how medicine was practiced by my predecessors, often through their own first person descriptions. I hope that readers will have a similar reaction and that this brief survey will make accessible for them a little-known aspect of Jewish history.

1

An Historical Perspective

This overview will serve as a frame of reference for the material to follow. Certain aspects of the general, medical, and Jewish history that are introduced here will be elaborated upon subsequently.

Biblical medicine's major contributions were in the area of hygiene and prevention. Diet; purification methods; cleanliness of the body, house, city, and camp; isolation of those with contagious disorders; and the importance of a weekly day of rest all were central themes.[1, 2]

Early Hebrew literature distinguished between the learned doctor (*rofe*) and the bloodletter (*umman*) and other medical craftsmen. It was understood that they had a right to adequate payment, for "a physician who works for nothing is worth nothing." Unlike Egyptian physicians, who generally were specialists, the first Jewish physicians were generalists who served all needs.

Of the 615 commandments of the law, 213 are of a medical nature, and the Talmud is replete with maxims related to health. Many of these are timeless, others of dubious value. They include the following:

- Drink boiled water and the devil will be powerless.
- He who leaves the lavatory without washing his hands creates danger.
- A physician should address his patient with animation, for the patient's eyes and heart are upon those who come to see him.
- A man of learning and discernment should not reside in a town without a physician.[3]

Julius Preuss, the esteemed authority on biblical and talmudic medicine, noted that only four people were explicitly given the title "physician" in the Talmud. However, he listed many talmudic examples of medical encounters, including *rofim* prescribing warm animal milk for a patient with consumption, curing a desperately ill Persian king with the milk of a lioness, treating a lovesick man by permitting him to see the object of his affection, an eye salve for a woman whose eyelashes fell out as a result of excessive crying, and so forth. *Rofim* drilled teeth, sucked out snakebites, healed wounds with herbs and dressings, and performed surgery, including brain surgery and amputations.[4]

A distinction between Greek medicine, as epitomized in the Hippocratic writings, and talmudic medicine was that the motives of the Greek physician, although altruistic and beneficent, were self-centered. Some Hippocratic ethical writings read like a primer for how to succeed professionally and achieve a good reputation. Conversely, the principal concern of the talmudic rabbis was that the physician should act in accordance with God's will in order to maintain the patient's welfare. Judaism holds that every moment of life is sacred and to preserve it is a religious duty.[5]

A major contribution of Hippocrates (fifth century B.C.E.), "The Father of Medicine," was to displace magic and pagan religion as the basis of medicine in favor of rational observation. The Greeks were superb diagnosticians, and their understanding of health was as a natural harmony of elements that could be restored by close attention to diet and life-style, akin to today's so-called "holistic" medicine. This afforded a basis for medical practice, but the Hippocratic approach fell into disfavor until it was reenergized and refined by Galen (c. 129–199 C.E.). Galen's influence was dominant for nearly fifteen hundred years, first in the Middle East and then throughout Europe, until it finally was challenged during the scientific renaissance of the sixteenth century.[6, 7, 8]

The numerous references to medical matters contained in the Bible and the Talmud were presented in a religious context. As a result, Jewish medicine, with its sensitive humane insights, had only an indirect influence on the development of medical practice in the general community. Indeed, Jewish physicians who lived during the period of Islamic rule substantially practiced medicine according to the Galenic system, albeit they regarded their vocation as being spiritually endowed and not merely an ordinary profession. A medieval rabbi wrote that "one should not try any of the medicines, prescriptions, or exorcisms recommended in the Talmud because no one today knows how they should be applied. If they should be tried nevertheless and found ineffective, the words of our sages would be exposed to ridicule."[9]

European medicine was stagnant during the Middle

Ages and dominated by a Catholic Church that was hostile to science and fixated upon the world to come. Scientific investigation and experimentation were unknown and undesired. Compared to classical medicine, the great service of the Church was that it undertook to take care of the sick regardless of their ability to pay. In fact, Jewish physicians had long adhered to the biblical teaching, "You should open your hand to your brother, to the needy and the poor."

Monastic medicine provided few original scientific ideas and substantially relied upon folk remedies. Beyond the Church, medicine was practiced mostly by Jews throughout the Middle Ages. Writing in 1845, a French historian said, "The Jews became almost the sole physicians of Europe . . . almost the only persons who knew how to treat disease with some system, from the advantages derived from the works of antiquity."[10]

That advantage was their reading and language skill. It is generally acknowledged that the major Jewish contribution during the medieval period was as translators and transmitters of Greek medical manuscripts, first to the Islamic and later to the Christian worlds, and to serve as intermediaries between those two hostile realms. By the thirteenth century, probably most of the hundreds of translators of Arabic texts into Latin were Jews working chiefly in Sicily, Spain, Provence, and North Italy. When the monks became familiar with classical and Arabic medicine, Galen's influence became dominant in Europe, as it already was in the Orient.

Medicine slowly began to break away from the Church, and education no longer was the exclusive province of the clergy. Previously, students had learned by working with experienced physicians, but from the ninth century on medical education began to become institutionalized. There is evidence that Salerno, recognized as the best of the new medical schools, and later, Montpellier, were founded with the help of Jews and employed medical compendiums and lists of prescriptions written by Jewish authors such as Shabbatai Donnolo and Isaac Israeli.[11]

The Arabs had conquered much of Spain in 711 C.E., and members of the small liberated Sephardic Jewish community soon became integrated into the dominant society and were permitted to practice medicine. The golden age for Jewish physicians in Spain spanned the ninth through twelfth centuries. Although they relied upon medical practice to earn a living, as learned men, in addition to Torah they also were fully conversant with Arabic culture and skilled in poetry, astronomy, mathematics, and philosophy. Famous Sephardic rabbis who also were physicians included Abraham Ibn Ezra (1089–1167), Nachmanides (1194–1267), Gersonides (1288–1344), and, of course, Maimonides (1135–1204).[12]

During the twelfth and thirteenth centuries, there was a resurgence of Christian control over Iberia, and Jewish fortunes began to decline. Some Jewish physicians continued to enjoy the protection and support of the reigning monarchs, but with increasing religious intolerance, many began to flee to safer places in southern France, Holland, Italy, North Africa, and Turkey. The brain drain became a deluge during what historian Barbara Tuchman called "the calamitous 14th century," when the Black Death (bubonic plague) of 1348 to 1350 wiped out nearly one-third of Europe's population. Jews were accused of well poisoning in order "to kill and destroy the whole of Christendom and have lordship over all the world."[13]

Among many bans that the Church initiated to isolate the Jews was prohibiting doctors from caring for Christians lest they exert too strong an influence over their minds. Paracelsus (1493–1541), one of the most influential physicians, articulated the intolerance of the period when he said, "As regards medicine, the Jews of old boasted greatly, and they still do, and they are not ashamed of the falsehood; they claim that they are the oldest and first physicians, and indeed they are the foremost among all the other nations, the foremost rascals that is."[14]

Nevertheless, kings and princes, popes and prelates continued to use Jewish physicians when their own health was in jeopardy, and many believed that it was essential to be of Jewish descent in order to be a skilled physician. In 1460 a Franciscan monk bemoaned the number of Jewish court physicians: "For many of the Jews, seeing how the Christians neglected the study . . . of medicine, worked with all their force to perfect the art, so that the temporal lords, nay—and that is the thing to weep over—the ecclesiastical prelates set great store by them, to such an extent that hardly one of them is to be found who does not harbor some devil of a Jew doctor."[15, 16]

With the Inquisition, a large proportion of Spanish and Portuguese Jews converted to Christianity and were called *conversos* or New Christians. Some of them were "crypto-Jews," so-called *marranos*, who secretly practiced their former religion. Others fled to lands of greater tolerance and safety. Then, with the final expulsion of Jews from Spain (1492), a tide of Sephardic immigration began to southern France, Italy, Turkey, and much more distant places, including India and the Americas. The less medically sophisticated Ashkenazim of northern Europe already were in flight to the east, particularly to Poland, for as Rabbi Moses Isserles later said, "Better to live on dry bread and in peace in Poland than remain in better conditions in more dangerous lands."

For some young men, a relatively safe haven existed in northern Italy at the University of Padua, which in the sixteenth century was recognized as being the best medical school in Europe. In Padua, there was a confluence of Sephardic and Ashkenazic emigres, as well as itinerant students from all over Europe who were imbued with an appetite for learning that characterized the Renaissance. The Jewish students absorbed new scientific and cultural ideas and when they returned to their native lands or continued on their migrations disseminated these, thereby contributing to what would become the Jewish Enlightenment (*haskalah*).

The medical curriculum in Padua introduced the method of bedside clinical teaching in hospitals and combined arts and science so that its graduates were sophisticated in many fields. Initially, the faculty was staunchly loyal to the Galenic tradition; their ultimate goal was to practice medicine in the manner of the ancients. However, the sixteenth century was a time of intellectual ferment and a new humanistic spirit prompted some daring souls like Galileo and Copernicus to consider new possibilities, generally at great personal risk. A medical renaissance was emerging, and the infallibility of Galen, "the perfect physician," now began to be challenged. Paracelsus concluded that the body was a chemical machine and popularized the use of minerals rather than plant-derived medicines. In 1543, the same year that Copernicus introduced his revolutionary theory about the nature of the universe, Vesalius published the first textbook of human anatomy. In it, Vesalius added to every Latin term its Hebrew equivalent in order that the Christian students should understand what was meant by the Latin terms.

Jews practiced medicine relatively freely in the cities and towns of Italy from the fifth century on, particularly in Rome, and many achieved fame as court physicians or authors of medical works. At first they obtained their knowledge by studying medical texts and by serving as apprentices, but beginning in the early sixteenth century the majority of Jewish physicians received their training in universities. At first it was difficult for Jews to receive the doctor's degree since it was conferred by the local bishop as a religious ceremony. However, later the Venetian Republic appointed a special official to confer the doctoral degree upon candidates of other faiths.

Sometimes medical dynasties continued the family tradition for several generations, and many Italian Jewish doctors also were rabbis and community leaders. The physicians were integrated into the Renaissance society more than any other Jewish class. However, with the Counter Reformation, a determined effort was made to drive the Jewish physicians out of practice. The medieval regulations, which forbade them to attend Christian patients, were renewed and implemented. In 1581, a bull issued by Pope Gregory XIII prohibited Jews from treating Christians and put an end to the golden age of Jewish medicine in Italy.[17, 18]

Nevertheless, Jewish students continued to travel to Padua and other Italian cities for more than two hundred years, since they continued to be denied entry into most European medical schools. Graduates of Italian medical schools practiced throughout Europe but everywhere were persecuted, insecure, and unable to participate in research or teaching. The nineteenth century bibliographer Moritz Steinschneider listed the names of 2,168 Jewish physicians who practiced from the Dark Ages until the eighteenth century. No doubt there were many more of less prominence whose names were unknown.

The largest concentration of Jews was in Poland, which in the eighteenth century was partitioned three times by its hostile neighbors (Russia, Prussia, and Austro–Hungary), disappearing altogether from the political map in 1795, not to reemerge until 1918. The largest remnant, and with it the largest number of Jews, fell to Russia, which contained its new citizens in a nearly four-hundred-thousand-square-mile appendage on its western border known as the Pale of Settlement. By the end of the nineteenth century, nearly 5 million Jews were concentrated in the Russian Pale.

Peter the Great had imported 125 trained foreign physicians to serve the needs of the military and in 1706 founded the first Russian hospital, but medical practice in Russia was primitive and lagged behind the rest of Europe. A French tourist, the Marquise de Custine, visited "Eternal Russia" in 1839 and observed that "the most able of those doctors of the princes are far inferior to the least known among the medical men of our own hospitals," and if a stranger falls sick in Russia, "his best plan is to consider himself among savages and to leave everything to nature."[19] But even in the more sophisticated West, the mainstays of medical treatment continued to be cupping, bleeding, purging, and toxic doses of mercury.

The nadir of Jewish medical fortunes occurred during the seventeenth and early eighteenth centuries, after which conditions began to improve with Austria's Act of Tolerance in 1782 and France's Declaration of the Rights of Man in 1789. New professional opportunities gradually opened up, but emancipation arrived much later in the Russian Pale, where Jews were not permitted to attend medical school until the 1860s. Even then, the good times were short-lived, for with the assassination of the relatively benevolent Czar Alexander II in 1881, a grim new government policy was initiated to address "the Jewish question"—one-third conversion, one-third emigration, and one-third starvation. Alternating between hope and despair and terrified by officially sanctioned pogroms, the Russian Jews began their mass exodus, especially to America.

Those who lived in more favorable circumstances in western Europe were able to participate in mainstream cultural and scientific affairs. Secular learning became a substitute for religion for many and some either became totally assimilated or converted out. To what extent their worldly success was attributable to a residue of forgotten or repressed cultural or religious influence is problematic, but increasingly the medical profession began to be dominated by Jews. By 1890 Jews constituted nearly half of the renowned medical faculty of Vienna University and until the start of World War I, they made up about half of Vienna's doctors when the general Jewish population constituted only about 9 percent of the total.[20]

For much of the recorded history of medicine, physicians had few treatments that could alter the outcome of disease, but the nineteenth century was a period of increased experimentation and refinement of diagnosis because of more precise instruments of measurement, flourishing of allied sciences, and increasing subdivision of medicine. Anesthesia was discovered and microorganisms were now understood to be important causes of disease. Bernard, Virchow, Pasteur, Semmelweis, Koch, and Lister were among the leaders of scientific progress. In the past, Jewish physicians had been more involved in the practice than the theory of medicine, but in post Enlightenment Germany they underwent a metamorphosis and actively participated in the first ranks. Now for the first time Jews were included in the pantheon of scientists, particularly in Germany. Barany, Breuer, Brill, Cohnheim, Einthoven, Henle, Kaposi, Landsteiner, Politzer, Romberg, Schick, Warburg, Wasserman, Weigert, Widal, and Zondek all are names that are still familiar today as major contributors to medical research.

The following chapters will develop the story in greater detail.

2

Early Jewish Opinions of Physicians

Honor a physician according to thy need of him
With the Honors due unto him.

Ben Sira (Ecclesiasticus 38:1–4)

Jewish opinion of physicians throughout history has generally been favorable. Indeed, the Talmud enjoins Jews against living in a city that lacks a doctor (*Sanhedrin* 17b). Judaism always has been preoccupied with health. The Bible and Talmud contain specific advice about prevention of disease, and more than a third of the 613 commandments concern health. Bodily cleanliness is thought to lead to spiritual purity, and since man is considered to be only a tenant in his body and not to have title, he doesn't have the right to abuse his health and is obliged to seek medical care.

Health and disease emanate from the same source. "I kill and I make alive; I wound and I heal," said God to Moses, and those who minister to the health of others are messengers of God and execute his will (Deuteronomy 32–39). *Pikuach Nefesh*, saving life, is a fundamental principle that suspends all religious laws—except

13

prohibitions against idolatry, unchastity, and unjustified bloodshed—even if the life saved might be of short duration or the outlook poor. Because of this, the opinions of physicians were critical if only to prognosticate about the possibility of saving life.

Moses assigned the priests the job of preventing contagious disease, but they didn't perform the same functions as physicians. Joseph employed physicians to embalm Jacob (Genesis 50:2), and in Exodus we read, "If men strive together and one smites another and he keepeth his bed . . . he shall pay for the loss of his time and shall cause him to be thoroughly healed."

Some priests discouraged the people from receiving health advice outside the temples, and an antagonistic relationship is implied in the biblical story of King Asa's terminal illness: "And in the thirty and ninth year of his reign, Asa was diseased in his feet; his disease was exceedingly great; yet in his disease he sought not to the Lord, but to the physicians. And Asa slept with his fathers and died in the one and fortieth year of his reign" (2 Chronicles 16:12–13).

Tension between science and religion has characterized much of Jewish history. In the thirteenth century, emerging mystical study of the Kabbalah was in direct conflict with the rationalistic approach championed by Maimonides. In 1305, the chief rabbi of Barcelona banned study of Greek philosophy and science for anyone under the age of twenty-five with the exception of medical science:

Woe to mankind because of the insult to the Torah!
For they have strayed far from it. . . .
No man under twenty-five shall study the books that
    the Greeks have written on religious philosophy and
    the natural sciences. . . .

Medicine, though one of the natural sciences,
Has not been included in our general prohibition
Because the Torah permits the physician to heal.[1]

Some of the early physicians viewed the study of
nature as a religious obligation, believing that studying
the visible world was equivalent to contemplating a
rabbinic text. This is well exemplified by Isaac Cardozo
(c. 1615–1680), who wrote, "We shall investigate nature and its founder, so that from the world and its multitude of things, as if by a ladder, with enlightened and
instructed mind, we may be lifted to God its maker; for
His creatures are the ladder by which we ascend to God,
the organ with which we praise God, and the school in
which we learn God."[2]

Although the Talmud had acknowledged that disease and its cure ultimately are in the hands of God,
physicians were understood to have a legitimate role as
God's agents and, therefore, they were esteemed. Conversely, a harsh epigram, attributed to Rabbi Judah HaNasi
(*Mishnah Kiddushin* IV, 14), "The best of physicians is
fit for *Gehenna* [Hell]" provoked much discussion through
the ages. According to the famous medieval commentator Rashi, physicians were censured for two reasons:
overconfidence in their craft, which resulted in their trusting in it instead of trusting in God, and commercializing
their profession to the extent that they sometimes failed
to attend the poor. Indeed, death of the neglected poor
was considered tantamount to homicide.[3]

Another explanation offered by a fifteenth-century
Spanish physician, Ibn Verga, was that the physician
should always see *Gehenna* opened before him lest he
cause the death of anyone whose health was entrusted
to him. He must carefully consider the treatment and
its consequences or else risk being sent to the nether-

world. Seventeenth-century Italian physician and tal-
mudist Isaac Lampronti suggested that the epigram spe-
cifically censured surgeons who, without the advice of
a good diagnostician, performed operations that caused
death.

The contemporary Jewish medical historian Dr. Fred
Rosner, who has studied the many interpretations of the
Gehenna epigram, suggests that it was never understood
as a denunciation of the conscientious practitioner. He
offers the following list for whom the curse was intended:

> those who are overly confident in their craft.
> those who are guilty of commercializing the profession.
> those who lie and deceive as do quacks.
> those who fail to acknowledge God as the true Healer of
> the sick.
> those who fail to consult with colleagues or medical texts
> when appropriate.
> those who perform surgery without heeding proper advice
> from diagnosticians.
> those who fail to heal the poor and thus indirectly cause
> their death.
> those who fail to try hard enough to heal their patients.
> those who consider themselves the best in their field.
> those who fail to conduct themselves in an ethical and
> professional manner.[4]

3

Medical Oaths
and Aphorisms

The first Jewish physician about whom anything is known was Asaph HaRofe. In fact, all we know about his personal life is that he lived sometime between the third and seventh centuries C.E. in the Middle East, probably in Syria. Asaph was the first to translate Greek medical literature into Hebrew. The Book of Asaph (*Sefer Asaph HaRofe*) summed up medical knowledge of the period and demonstrated that the contemporary understanding of pathology was primitive although there were flashes of modern insight.[1, 2]

For example, Asaph described meningitis as "a bad spirit" and related how at the time a woman comes from the river or the privy or when she discharges feces and does not wash her hands and gives bread or milk to her son, "there is a bad ghost, Saturn by name, that seizes youths and bends and breaks their necks. . . . There is no cure, but to burn with fire." Today we call those bad spirits microbes. Asaph also was among the first to anticipate hereditary disease when he described how sometimes "the humor and illnesses are already on the sperm and are transmitted to the embryo."[3]

Asaph taught medical students in one of the Syrian schools and would have them join him in a covenant that resembled the famous Oath of Hippocrates, which had been written some 500 to 1,000 years earlier. Asaph's oath was more a statement of medical morality, Hippocrates' more a guide on how to succeed professionally. The Oath of Hippocrates began with the physician swearing to Apollo and other gods and goddesses, while Asaph and his students pledged allegiance to "the One God, the Lord of Israel and the whole world, the true Healer of the sick."

Unlike the Greeks, the Jewish oath strongly prohibited sorcery and idol worship. Physicians were expected to provide care for the poor free of charge for the sake of charity, for "thou shall not harden your heart against the poor and needy, but heal them." Among Asaph's other admonitions to his students were the following: "Beware of causing death to anyone by administering the juices of poisonous roots. Do not administer to an adulterous wife an abortifacient drug. Let not the beauty of woman arouse in thee the passion of adultery. Divulge not any secret entrusted to thee, and do no act of injury or of harm for any price."

The Jewish medical ethics encoded in the Oath of Asaph included the sanctity and dignity of human life, opposition to superstition and irrational cures, rigid dietary restraints, and sexual morality. Whereas observation of the Hippocratic Oath would bring success and fame, following its precepts was entirely voluntary. Conversely, the Jewish physician was obliged to comply because the text was within a religious framework based on biblical law. Failure to comply would result in loss of God's support because "the Lord is with you as long as you are with him."

Another early Middle Eastern Jewish physician, Isaac Judaeus, also known as Isaac ben Solomon Israeli, was born in Egypt before 850 C.E. and distinguished himself as an oculist and physician. He studied in Bagdad and was said to be indifferent to wealth or personal advancement. In 909 C.E. he became court physician to the caliph of Kairwan (Tunisia). The caliph enjoyed his learning and wit, and under his patronage, Isaac's power and fame grew. He wrote medical books concerning urinoscopy, dietetics, pharmacology, and fever, never married, and when asked whether he would not be happy to have children to live after him, replied, "I shall leave my book on fever as my posterity."[4]

One Arabic scholar remarked that Isaac "lived a hundred years and composed valuable works . . . which cannot be weighed in gold and silver." His works were written in Arabic but later were widely translated into Hebrew and Latin, and during the Middle Ages Isaac was cited as an authority of the rank of Hippocrates, Galen, and Rhazes. He particularly is remembered for his medical aphorisms, of which I list here only a few:

- Most illnesses are cured without the physician's help through the aid of nature.
- If you can cure the patient by dietary means, do not turn to drugs.
- Do not rely on cure-alls, for they depend mostly on ignorance and superstition.
- Try to ease the mind of the patient, encourage him to look forward to being cured, even if thou art not thyself convinced of it, for this will greatly strengthen his nature.

- It is fitting to the profession of a physician that he should be moderate in eating—that he should not become a debaucher or a glutton. It is a shame and a reproach if he suffer from tedious illness, for then the people will say, "How should he who cannot cure himself cure others?"
- Suffer not thy mouth to condemn when something happens to a physician, for everyone has his evil day. Let thy deeds praise thee, and seek not thine honor in another's shame.
- ·Fix the fee of thy patient when his disease is in its ascendency and most severe, for as soon as he is cured he will forget what service thou hast rendered.[5]

In his *Preparatory Instruction for Physicians*, Isaac wrote, "If you find a physician who is ready as soon as asked to give information about every disease and particularly to praise his own methods of treatment, you may regard him as a knave. . . . Too large a practice confuses the judgment of the physician and causes him to give mistaken directions."

Some six centuries after Isaac, a former Portuguese *marrano*, Amatus Lusitanus (1511–1568) now living in Italy (see chapter 7) wrote a medical oath that was much in the spirit of Hippocrates but distinctly from a Jewish perspective. Here are but a few excerpts:

I swear by God the Almighty and Eternal and by his holy Ten Commandments given on Mount Sinai by the hand of Moses the lawgiver, after the People of Israel had been freed from the bondage of Egypt, that I have never in my medical practice departed from what had been handed down in good faith to us and posterity; that I have never practiced deception, I have never overstated or made changes for the sake of gain. . . . I have not been desireful for the remuneration for medical services and have treated many without accepting any fee, but with none the less care. . . . Loftiness of station has never influenced me, and I have accorded the same care to the poor as to those of exalted rank. I have never produced disease. In stating my opinion, I have always told what I believed to be true. I have favored no druggist unless he excelled others in his skill in his art and in character. . . . I have been diligent and have allowed nothing to divert me from the study of good authors. I have endured the loss of private fortune and have suffered frequent and dangerous journeys and even exile with calmness and unflagging courage, as befits a philosopher. . . . I have published my medical works not to satisfy ambition, but that I might, in some measure, contribute to the furtherance of the health of mankind.[6]

In every century there were some Jewish physicians who had a strong sense of social and professional responsibility. Jacob Zahalon (1630–1693) of Rome was religiously devout and stressed the value of preaching in the synagogue. During an epidemic of plague when public places were closed, he preached out of the open window of a friend's house to the throngs in the street below. The Jewish ghetto was divided into three districts, each supervised by a physician, and Zahalon alone of the three survived. In all, about a fifth of Rome's Jewish population of four thousand succumbed. Zahalon's greatest medical work, *The Treasure of Life* (*Otzar HaHayyim*), published in 1683, was an encyclopedic summary of the medical knowledge of his day. He also composed a Physician's Prayer (1665) that he urged all physicians to recite at least once a week. In it he observed that medicine was a sacred calling. The physician merely treats and God cures: "Thou art the physician, not I. I am but as the clay

in the potter's hand. . . . I pray that I may discover the
secrets of Thy wonderful deeds and that I may know the
peculiar curative powers which Thou has placed in herbs
and minerals . . . and that through them I shall tell of Thy
might to all generations to whom Thy greatness shall
come." The following items are of particular interest
today:

- "And may my sustenance and that of my children and
  children's children come from Thy hands . . . and may
  it be in abundance so that I be not forced to take anything from the poor and sick, but on the contrary, that
  I may be able to give unto them what Thou hast be-
  stowed upon me."
- "I ask one favor of Thee, that Thou give strength to my
  memory so that when I go to visit a patient, Thou make
  known to me at once which cure will benefit him,
  whether I have studied it or not."
- "If there comes to me any patient whose allotted time
  is about to end and whose affliction is heavy, may it
  be Thy will I cause not the hastening of his death even
  by one second. Teach me to administer drugs so as to
  retain his soul within him until his fated hour arrives."[7,8]

Separated as they were by a millennium of history,
what was common to the oaths and aphorisms of Asaph
HaRofe, Isaac Israeli, Amatus Lusitanus, and Jacob Zahalon was their conviction that medical practice was a
moral undertaking, that the physician's hand was guided
by his Maker, and that physicians should conduct themselves in a responsible, altruistic, and dignified manner.

4

Maimonides, "The Eagle of Physicians"

At the end of the seventh century, the armies of Islam set out to conquer the world. The Iberian peninsula was captured, the Spanish Jewish community liberated, and a fertile era ensued during which Muslim, Christian, and Jewish cultures comingled. The zenith of Jewish integration into the mainstream was during the ninth and tenth centuries, when their intellectual and scientific center was the Andalusian capital Cordova. The medical profession was perhaps the single most important avenue of advancement for non-Muslims in Islamic society, and almost every caliph employed Jewish or Christian physicians.

Some Sephardic doctors achieved political power, notably Hasdai ibn Shaprut (915–970), who gave the caliph both medical and political advice and was an influential diplomat. Yehudah Halevi (1085–1145) was only a minor court physician but a major poet. He jested about his lowly status during a medical call to a harem:

They called me in but they did not call to me,
Among them, yet I was not one of them,
My visits were not those of a visitor:
They sought my skill but ignored my heart.[1]

Surely the most illustrious medieval Jewish physician in Arab lands was Moses Maimonides (Rambam). He was born in Cordova, Spain, in 1135, but when Moses was thirteen, his family fled from a fanatical invading Islamic group (the Almohades) and wandered for more than a decade before settling in Fostat, a suburb of Cairo. Within a few years both his father and brother died and it fell upon Maimonides to support the family. And so, at the age of thirty-three and already an acclaimed interpreter of Bible and Talmud, he embarked upon a career in medicine strictly for economic reasons.

Maimonides was a prolific medical writer and composed at least ten books that were written in Arabic for general consumption. His *Medical Aphorisms* contained twenty-five chapters and fifteen hundred maxims based mainly on Greek medical writings, particularly the works of Hippocrates and Galen. He wrote monographs on hemorrhoids, treatment of poisoning, and asthma, and his approach to treatment was always based upon common sense and personal observation.[2, 3, 4]

Maimonides emphasized prevention, good hygiene, fresh air, exposure to sun, drinking fresh water, preservation of food, good sewage, and moderation in drinking and lovemaking. He believed that a healthy body is necessary for a healthy soul and that a physician should understand the patient's personality and environment in addition to having technical knowledge. Regarding exercise, "Nothing is to be found that can subsitute for exercise in any way . . . (it) will expel the harm done by most of the bad regimes that most men follow."

In his *Medical Aphorisms*, Maimonides discussed the importance of nutrition in both health and disease. "We, the association of physicians, strive that foods should benefit and not [be consumed purely] for pleasure. . . . It is not for us to gorge ourselves with food like a dog when we are hungry, . . . even more important is that we not stretch our hand out to that which is placed or happens to be before us, especially sweets and the like, which are designated as 'gluttonous foods.'"[5]

Maimonides also counseled that chicken soup is an excellent food as well as medication and praised the efficacy of wine taken daily in moderation. He admitted that on rainy days he himself used to drink a small glass of white wine before going to bed and advised that wine is especially good for old people since it keeps them warm and helps their urination and digestion. All of this may be splendid advice, but it is more difficult to assess his suggestion that turtledoves increase memory, improve intellect, and sharpen the senses.

It is noteworthy that Maimonides' medical practice as a physician at the sultan's court was exhausting and sometimes demeaning. Consider the introduction to his monograph on the treatment of impotence, which was written for the hedonistic nephew of Saladin: "Our lord his majesty—may Allah [!] make his power last long! —ordered me to compose for him a treatise on behavior which would help to increase his sexual power, as he had mentioned that he had some hardship in this way . . . (the sultan) desires an augmentation (of sexual power) on account of the increasing number of female slaves."[6]

Maimonides complained that the demands of medical practice detracted from his study time, "for you know
how exacting and difficult is this profession for any
person of conscience." The following account, written
near the end of his life in a letter to his translator Samuel
Ibn Tibbon, who lived in France, describes Maimonides'
typical workday:

> I live in Fostat and the Sultan resides in Cairo; these
> two places are two Sabbath limits (about one and
> one-half miles) distant from each other. My duties to
> the Sultan are very heavy. I am obliged to visit him every
> day, early in the morning, and when he or any of
> his children or concubines are indisposed, I cannot
> leave Cairo but must stay during most of the day in
> the palace. It also frequently happens that one or two
> of the officers fall sick and I must attend to their heal-
> ing. Hence, as a rule every day, early in the morning
> I go to Cairo and even if nothing unusual happens
> there, I do not return to Fostat until the afternoon. Then
> I am famished but I find the antechambers filled
> with people, both Jews and gentiles, nobles and com-
> mon people, judges and policemen, friends and ene-
> mies—a mixed multitude who await the time of my
> return. I dismount from my animal, wash my hands,
> go forth to my patients and entreat them to bear with
> me while I partake of some light refreshment, the only
> meal I eat in twenty-four hours. Then I go attend
> to my patients and write prescriptions and directions
> for their ailments. Patients go in and out until night-
> fall, and sometimes, even as the Torah is my faith, until
> two hours and more into the night. I converse with
> them and prescribe for them even while lying down
> from sheer fatigue. When night falls, I am so exhausted
> that I can hardly speak. In consequence of this, no

Israelite can converse with me or befriend me except on the Sabbath.[7]

If overworked by his masters in court, Maimonides was admired by his peers and described as "the most distinguished physician of his time, both in theory and in practice." A Baghdad physician, Abd al-Latif, visited Cairo and described Maimonides as "the eagle of physicians." Another contemporary referred to him as "the physician of the century," and seven centuries later the famous Canadian physician Sir William Osler called him "the prince of physicians."

Maimonides railed against quackery and superstition and condemned the pseudoscience of astrology. He didn't blindly accept the teachings of others but wrote, "Don't believe anyone's theory without testing it yourself." And elsewhere, "There is a feeling among the educated men of our time and surely among the multitude. They do not examine a statement by its contents, but by its conformity to the statement of the previous author without having evaluated the former statement." Although he considered Galen a master in medical matters, he didn't completely accept his dogmatic authority and dared to point out inconsistencies in Galen's work.

Probably Maimonides should not be credited for the famous Physician's Prayer that tradition has attributed to him. Modern scholarship suggests that it was written in 1790 by Dr. Markus Herz of Berlin (1747–1803) (see chapter 11). In this century, Osler described the prayer as "one of the most precious documents of our profession, worthy to be placed beside the Hippocrates oath." Others have suggested that even if Maimonides was not its author, the prayer's form and spirit are in complete harmony with his other writings and for this reason one of the many versions of the Physician's Prayer is reproduced here:

O God, Thou hast formed the body of man with infinite goodness. Thou hast united in him immeasurable forces incessantly at work like so many instruments so as to preserve in its entirety this beautiful house containing his immortal soul, and these forces act with all the order and harmony imaginable. But if weakness or violent passion should disturb this harmony, these forces would act against one another and the body return to the dust whence it came. Thou sendest to man Thy messenger the disease which announces the approach of danger and bids him prepare to overcome them. The eternal Providence has appointed me to watch o'er the life and health of Thy creatures. May the love of my art actuate me at all times; may neither avarice nor thirst for glory or ambition for reputation engage my mind, for enemies of truth and philanthropy they could easily deceive me and make me forgetful of my lofty aim of doing good to Thy children. Endow me with strength of mind and heart so that both be always ready to serve the rich and the poor, the good and the wicked, friend and foe, and that I may never see in the patient anything else but a fellow creature in pain.

If physicians more learned than I wish to guide and counsel me, inspire me with confidence in, obedience toward, recognition of them, for the study of the science is great. It is not given to one man alone to see what others see. May I be moderate in everything, except in the knowledge of this science; as far as it is concerned, may I be insatiable in the desire to learn. Grant me strength and opportunity to always correct what I have acquired, to always extend its [medicine's] domain, for knowledge is immense and the spirit of man can also extend infinitely to daily enrich itself with new acquirements. Today he can discover his errors of yesterday, and tomorrow he may obtain new light on what he thinks himself sure of today. O God, Thou hast appointed me to watch o'er the health of Thy creatures; here am I ready for my vocation.[8]

5

The Perils of Court Life

Maimonides was an outstanding example of a court physician, but there were many others. From the thirteenth century on, nearly every pope and ruler in Italy had a Jewish medical attendant, for Jewish physicians were thought to have at their command vast stores of secret medical doctrine that was unknown to Christians. A professor in Leipzig lamented, "There is hidden in the literature of the Jews a treasure of medical lore so great that it seems incapable of being surpassed by any books in any other language. . . . And what prevents our Christian youths . . . who are taking up this profession from learning this language?"[1]

Indeed, gentile physicians were often despised and denounced because of their high fees and haughty airs. In about 1352 Petrarch advised the sick Pope Clement VI against trusting physicians:

I know that your bedside is beleaguered by doctors, and naturally this fills me with fear. Their opinions are always conflicting, and he who has nothing new to say suffers the shame of limping behind the others. . . . They learn their art at our expense, and even our death brings them experience; the physician alone has the right to kill with impunity. Oh, most Gentle Father, look upon their band as an army of enemies. Remember the warning epitaph which an unfortunate man had inscribed on his tombstone: "I died of too many physicians."[2]

Having been expelled from Germany after the Black Plague and later from Spain and Portugal, Jewish physicians were ubiquitous in European courts during the fifteenth and sixteenth centuries. Generally they were treated with favor, but if their efforts failed, or if they were suspected of spying or conspiracy, they were severely punished. For example, in 1490 a Venetian Jew named Master Leo (also referred to as Leon Zhidovin or "Leo the Jew") arrived in Moscow and rashly wagered his life that he could cure the eldest son of Czar Ivan III, who suffered from leg pains, with the following recorded result:

> The doctor began his treatment by giving the Prince simples to drink; he began to burn him about the body with glasses into which he poured boiling water; thereupon the Prince grew much worse and died. Leo, originally obnoxious as a Jew to all true believers, was doubly so as a foul sorcerer who had brought about the death of the heir to the throne. The forfeit to which he so boastfully bound himself was exacted to the full, and he was publicly executed six weeks after the death of his patient.[3]

In 1492, the same year that Jews were expelled from Spain, Jewish doctors may have played central roles in the deaths of two prominent Italians. The veracity of the following story is in doubt, but it was reported that when Pope Innocent VIII lay on his deathbed, too feeble to ingest anything other than woman's milk, a Jewish phyician, whose name is unknown, attempted a startling remedy—a blood transfusion! Three ten-year-old boys were chosen for the purpose and were paid a ducat each for their services. The boys died in the course of the experiment and the pope presumably obtained no benefit.[4]

In the very same year of 1492, Lorenzo the Magnificent also lay dying. He was visited by the monk Savonarola, who exhorted him to repent, but Lorenzo continued to fail. The Medici doctor, an old friend, was accused of gross incompetence and committed suicide when he realized the extent of his bungling. Then, the duke of Milan was informed of the seriousness of Lorenzo's condition and sent for the most eminent physician in his duchy—the Jew Lazzaro da Pavia. When he arrived at the Villa Medici, the doctor found Lorenzo to be in a critical condition and resorted to a potion of crushed pearls and precious gems. Lorenzo drank the concoction and died shortly afterward. Such was his reputation, however, that it was said if only "maestro Lazzero hebreo" had been called sooner, Lorenzo the Magnificent might have been saved. Indeed, there was widespread belief in the curative powers of precious stones among Jews and gentiles alike.[5]

A *marrano* court physician, Elijah Montalto, was born in Portugal in the late sixteenth century and christened Felipe Rodriguez. The details of his early life are unknown except that he married into a prominent *marrano* family distinguished for its well-known physicians. He achieved medical success and, in time, was sought after by royalty both in Italy and France. In 1606, Montalto formally avowed his Judaism, and when Queen Marie de Medici of France wrote to the pope to obtain special dispensation to be treated by the Jewish physician, Montalto insisted that he be permitted to practice his religion unencumbered. This was laudable, but he was not too pious to write the following justification in order to explain his violating the Sabbath by riding in a coach to visit his royal patients:

> I am feeble and ailing and my health is bad. Besides, if I walk a long distance on foot, as one is forced to do in the streets of Paris, I shall become more feeble, fatigued, and my health will suffer. In short, I have tried it many times and have found that it takes all my strength. . . . I do not desire to draw in the additional argument of personal dignity . . . what humiliation if the physician of the King and Queen walks afoot in the streets of Paris! And besides the streets are full of mud. It is impossible for anyone to walk without covering his clothes and his boots with dirt, as all know who have been here. And it is contemptuous to present oneself before the King with soiled clothes.

After Montalto's death, the queen ordered that his body be taken to Amsterdam for a religious burial in a Jewish cemetery, which then was impossible in France.[6]

Moshe Fiszel was born into a wealthy Cracow family of "court Jews." Having completed his rabbinical studies in Poland, he went to Padua to obtain his doctor of medicine degree. On his return, King Sigismund I exempted him from all taxes paid by Jewish residents and in 1532 appointed him chief rabbi of the Jewish community of Kazimierz. He had a brilliant career that came to an abrupt end when he was falsely accused of encouraging

the conversion of Christians to Judaism and of participation in a ritual child murder. He was arrested, thrown
into prison, tortured, and died shortly after his release.[7]

Perhaps the most prominent Jewish physician in
Russia at the time was Antonio Ribeira Sanchez (1699–
1783), a *marrano* who was born in Portugal, studied
medicine in Salamanca, and fled to Holland to escape
persecution. In Leyden he was a pupil of the great Dutch
physician Hermann Boerhaave, and when the Russian
empress regent Anna asked Boerhaave to recommend
three physicians from among his pupils for positions in
her state, Sanchez was the first named. He served as
chief municipal physician in Moscow, moved to St.
Petersburg in 1733, and distinguished himself in the field
of public health and particularly in the study of syphilis.
A gifted physician, he was credited with curing Empress
Catherine II of a "serious illness" (given her well-known
proclivities, possibly syphilis) and was awarded many
distinctions, which inevitably caused envy and jealousy.
In 1747, Sanchez's *marrano* origins became known and
he began to receive death threats. He asked for his release and moved to Paris, where he practiced medicine
among the poor and lived in poverty until Catherine II
learned of his condition and granted him a life pension
of one thousand rubles annually.[8]

A final example of the hazards of being a court
physician is the story of Rodrigo Lopez. Born in Portugal
in 1525, he was captured by Sir Francis Drake and brought
to England. He became physician to the earl of Leicester
and was suspected of assisting the earl in disposing of
his enemies by poisoning. Later he became physician to
Queen Elizabeth, who granted him a monopoly in im-
porting anise seed and sumac into England. He amassed
a fortune but in the process made many enemies. After

thirty-five years of service, in 1594 he was accused of conspiracy against the queen, confessed when put on the rack, and was hanged, drawn, and quartered. The case attracted much attention and a great deal was written about the unfairness of his trial. It has been suggested that Lopez was the prototype of Shylock in Shakespeare's *Merchant of Venice*.[9]

6

Black Bile
and Black Death
in Renaissance Italy

From the death of Galen in 199 C.E. to the rebirth of medicine in mid-sixteenth century, the dominant theory of health and sickness was the highly structured Galenic system, which depended on a balance of many factors that were thought to affect bodily function, including air, climate, food and drink, sleep and waking, evacuation, and so on. All disorders were attributed to unbalance (dyscrasia) of one or more of the four humors—blood, phlegm, choler (yellow bile), and melancholer (black bile)—and variable mixtures of these determined an individual's complexion or temperament. Curing a patient involved restoring normal balance through a combination of purges, emetics, or bloodletting and adherence to dietetic and hygienic principles. It was believed that nature heals and rest and diet were emphasized. Also, it didn't hurt to introduce some astrological medicine and magical healing techniques. Such "therapeutic eclecticism" may have been effective for some conditions but surely not for scourges such as bubonic plague, which was known as the Black Death.

Manipulation and management of all of these variables by the medieval physician was called "regimen" and was highly individualized and not universally applicable. Gradually, however, there were conceptual changes and a greater reliance on medicine to cure the sick rather than to preserve health. Total life manipulation was too slow to achieve an effect, and medical or magical treatment definitely was more profitable and widely applicable. The Jewish physician had the additional burden of reconciling these concerns with his natural ambivalence about astrology and superstition as well as possible conflicts with talmudic dietary advice.[1]

All of this is well illustrated by the practice of Amatus Lusitanus (1511–1568). Born Juan Roderigo to *marrano* parents, he studied medicine and surgery in Salamanca and later escaped the Portuguese Inquisition. In spite of his persecution, he picked the name Amatus (love) for himself and, in spite of the fact that Portugal had driven him out, took the surname Lusitanus after the province in which he was born. He lived a harried, peripatetic life and didn't begin to practice Judaism openly until he came to Salonika in 1558.[2]

Amatus was a prolific medical writer and an astute clinical observer whose major research concerned the anatomy of the veins. In one anatomy lecture, he dissected twelve cadavers in front of his audience in order to demonstrate the function of the valves of the venous system. His reasoning was flawed by modern standards, but he was bold enough to dispute the findings of Vesalius and he anticipated the later work of Harvey.

Amatus published a seven-volume collection of his most interesting cases (*Centuriae curationum*), each volume containing one hundred case reports that provide a remarkable insight into medical practice of the time. In one he related the story of a young girl who suffered from a chronic digestive disorder. Her father was a Hebrew teacher who had among his students a Jewish physician, whom he asked for medical advice. The doctor agreed to treat the girl by administering an enema, but unfortunately she died an hour later. The father started what today would be a malpractice suit, and Amatus was called as an expert witness to defend the doctor. In his testimony he commented that it is well known that the Jews eat "melancholic food" that produces flatulence; therefore, they are frequently troubled by digestive disturbances.

He expanded upon this phenomenon in another case, that of the noted Hebrew scholar and physician Azariah dei Rossi of Mantua. They met in a Roman bookshop, where Azariah consulted with his colleague about his own symptoms, which included indigestion, insomnia, and chest pressure. Amatus attributed them to melancholia and recalled that Hippocrates, Galen, and Maimonides all had written that those who chronically suffer from fear and sadness develop black bile. Since all Hebrews are black-biled, Azariah, who was "extremely studious and zealously occupied with his medical work," was no exception.

Amatus's treatment for black bile was first to avoid foggy, moist weather, then to concentrate on the diet. Drink fruit juice mildly cooked, not too rich so as neither to cause flatulence nor constipation. Eat white bread—light, well-kneaded, and covered with caraway seeds to avoid flatulence. Avoid unleavened bread or, during the feast of Passover, it should be prepared with sugar and eggs so as to make it lighter and more digestible. Avoid cold meat, as is common among the Jews, namely, beef, smoked and strongly salted meat, goose, duck, and the like. Permitted are squabs but not quail or turtledoves. Most vegetables and fruits are acceptable, including "melopepones, vulgarly called melons, which quite without reason are now so unpopular."

The remainder of the regimen included massage, rest, and advice not to study at night because it is "harmful and contrary to nature." Of less appeal to modern sensibility is bloodletting. Amatus noted that since the patient was emaciated and weak, venesection from the elbow would be dangerous, so "two leeches should be applied to the veins at the anus called hemorrhoidal to withdraw the black humor." He concluded that having followed this course of treatment for four months, the patient's strength increased to that of a boxer.

A pandemic of Black Death wiped out much of Europe's population in 1347–1348 and sporadic epidemics continued for several centuries due to spread of the bacillus by insects and rodents as a result of poor sanitation. The physician who visited the sick during the plague wore long protective gowns of smooth material or leather, the color of which was red or black. He also wore gloves and a mask over his face; the mask had special openings for the eyes and a beak in which fragrant substances or fumigants were stored. The pulse was felt with a special wand in order to avoid direct contact with the patient.[3]

Popular prejudice laid the blame for plague epidemics on deliberate poisoning, and this fantasy was used as a pretext to persecute the Jews. David Ruderman, in his detailed study of the Italian physician-scholar Abraham Yagel (1553–1623), describes how plague was understood and treated during an epidemic. Yagel was well schooled in Galenic theory and also was aware of emerging new theories concerning astrologic and cosmic influences on health. In addition, he was influenced by the magic and mysticism contained in the Kabbalah, and he attempted to integrate all of these—science, astronomy, and religion—into a unified system.[4]

Consider Yagel's therapeutic approach for a patient with plague: As with any illness, the patient should first ask God's forgiveness and then seek out a physician to effectuate a cure. In turn, the physician should offer prayers to God, by whose agency he is able to heal. After cursory examination and diagnosis, blood is drawn, "since the majority of human illnesses arise from the increase of the blood when bloodletting is not performed at the appropriate time." Purgatives to weaken the power of the illness and healthful food and drink also are prescribed. Concerning the three causes of plague, the earthly is due to emanation of poisonous gas from the ground, particularly for those who are susceptible because of humoral imbalance. A celestial cause relates to the position of the stars, and a divine cause is God's revenge against those who transgress religious law. Having identified the causes, the treatment addresses each in turn. For the material cause, a long list of practical advice is offered ranging from proper diet, to purification of water and air, to avoidance of "overheating" through excessive sexual activity and rich foods. For the celestial cause, incense is burned and talismans and incantations employed according to kabbalistic convention. Then, on the divine level, God's forgiveness is asked through prayer and fasting.

Yagel was one of a small but growing number of Jewish physicians in sixteenth-century Italy who were receptive to new ideas and attempted to reconcile them with their religious beliefs. The focus for this medical renaissance was in Padua.

7

Padua's Unique
Influence

In the sixteenth century students flocked to the University of Padua because of the excellence of its bedside teaching, which was led by capable clinicians. The curriculum emphasized classical and contemporary learning, and most physicians graduated with a combined degree in medicine and philosophy. The first Jew graduated from Padua in 1409; between 1517 and 1619 more than eighty others obtained medical degrees and hundreds more followed until well into the eighteenth century.[1, 2]

Padua was not the only Italian university to accept Jews, but it protected them from violence and illegal measures, and when in 1588 Pope Gregory XIII forbade Jews to practice medicine except among themselves, it was the only Italian university to maintain a tolerant attitude. Jewish students were allowed to wear the black beret of their colleagues rather than the yellow one required of other Jews. Nevertheless, they were required to pay double the tuition and also were burdened with special taxes, including a requirement to deliver 170 pounds of sweetmeat to Christian students upon graduation.[3]

Some Jewish students combined their medical studies with learning at Padua's famous talmudic academy. Many were ill prepared to meet the prerequisites of admission or lacked sufficient knowledge of Latin, the language of instruction, and had to take preparatory work. Their desire for medical education often met with disapproval from their religious leaders back home, who resisted secular education, and in some cases the high cost of their studies in Padua was underwritten by members of the Polish aristocracy. In return they agreed to return and serve their patrons as family physicians for a limited period.

Owing to the recent invention of the printing press, there was an information explosion in the sixteenth century, and foreign students became exposed to the latest cultural ideas as well as to the classics. When these cosmopolitan physicians returned to their native lands, they were intellectually transformed and disseminated the new thinking; no doubt, they had a substantial influence.

Joseph Shelomoh Delmedigo (1591–1655) came from an influential family of physicians, rabbis, and scholars on the island of Crete. He began his medical studies at age fifteen in Padua, where he also studied mathematics under Galileo. He had a broad range of knowledge and was a prolific writer on a variety of subjects. During this period of transition both in Jewish life and in science, he was a rationalist who also was intrigued by Jewish mysticism (Kabbalah). Relying on both theory and practice, he was among those physicians who were beginning to abandon the Galenic and Hippocratic theories and wrote that if one wished to formulate a clear idea of any specific problem, he should examine the prevalent opinion, but through his own sense.[4]

Delmedigo traveled extensively, and in 1620 he settled in Vilna, where he entered general practice. He gained popularity with the nobility and served for a time as personal physician to Prince Radziwill, practicing by day and studying science and Talmud most of the night. During the week he made rounds in the neighboring villages, and on the Sabbath he lectured in synagogue. Delmedigo disdained the teaching methods employed in Jewish schools of Poland and Lithuania and deplored the dirt and filth that he found in the ghettos. Alone and unhappy, finding neither the intellectual climate nor the harsh northern conditions to his liking, he moved again, this time to Frankfurt, where he agreed to serve as physician for the Jewish community. His contract, written in Hebrew, declared, ". . . we have appointed the competent physician, the learned Joseph b. Elia (Delmedigo) for five years to take care of every sickness—may it be far from us!" As described in Marcus's study of communal sick care in Germany, he was to take care of the poor without charge, was not to leave the city without permission, and could not refuse to treat a Jew, whether rich or poor. Initially he was exempted from taxes but would have to pay his assessment if he became wealthy. A fee schedule was established and haggled over during the subsequent years and Delmedigo remained in Frankfurt until 1645, when he moved on to Prague, where he died in 1655.[5]

Another graduate of Padua was Toviah Cohen (Toviah Rofe, 1652–1729), who was born in Metz and was the last in a line of prominent physicians. His father was a rabbinic scholar and upon his death, Toviah and his

mother moved to Cracow, where he studied at the
yeshivah. He and a friend, Gabriel Felix of Brody, decided to go abroad to study medicine. They worked
briefly in Danzig with a local doctor, but recognizing
the need for more formal training, they appealed to the
grand elector of Brandenburg to allow them to study at
the University of Frankfurt. The prince granted their re-
quest despite his counselors, who advised him to reject
the Jews on the grounds that "such people" were sus-
picious and might desecrate the Christian religion. The
hostility against Jews was typified by a statement by the
medical faculty of Vienna University (1610): "The Jews
are bound by their law to destroy the life of every tenth
Christian patient by drugs." Cohen and Felix were among
the first Jews to be accepted into a European medical
school, but faculty members attempted to persuade them
to convert to Christianity. Tired of the countless religious
disputes, they transferred to Padua, where Toviah matriculated in 1681.[6]

Toviah Cohen found the intellectual climate in
Padua conducive and broadening. Referring to the new
chemical philosophy introduced by Paracelsus, which
was then beginning to supplant Galen's humoral theory
of disease, he wrote of the flowering of "a new medicine which dwells in the bosom of the physician of our
time." After completing his studies in 1683, Cohen practiced in Cracow for several years and then moved on to
Constantinople, where he served as court physician for
five successive sultans. He acquired a considerable fortune, and at the age of sixty-two he retired from the court
and moved again, this time to Jerusalem, where he lived
for fourteen years and concentrated on Torah study.

Cohen's major book, the encyclopedic *Maaseh
Tuviah* (*Toviah's Tales*), which was written in Hebrew

and first published in 1707, contained chapters on theology, astronomy, pharmacy, botany, hygiene, venereal diseases, and chemistry. His remedies included laxatives, emetics, cupping, and bleeding, and he criticized those who believed in miracle cures and superstition. Cohen lamented, "Medicine is a very simple science, if it is practiced by charlatans. On the other hand, it is a very difficult one when practiced by a schooled physician." He noted that

in no land is the practice of summoning up devils and spirits by means of the kabbalistic abracadabra so prevalent and the belief in dreams and visions so strong as in Poland. ... Those who permit themselves to be treated by a physician who has not studied the entire theory of medicine can be likened to those who, when journeying on an ocean, entrust their fate to the winds; sometimes the winds drive the ship to its destination, but more often they cause it to sink. Those who think any kind of practice makes a good physician are sadly mistaken.[7]

Toviah Cohen was a transitional figure between the classical medicine of Galen and Hippocrates and the new scientific developments of his time. He wrote, "I do not wish, beloved reader, to force you to follow in a rigorous way my teachings, and to urge you to go in the ways of modern physicians without deviating to right or left; but it is true that the method which modern physicians use with constancy and reflective analysis has led them to new discoveries ... thus they have enlightened us so that they could establish in our time a practical method of medicine."

Despite Dr. Cohen's progressive attitude, he was nevertheless a product of his time. For example, he was the first to describe a scalp condition called "plica polonica," a tangled, ropelike mass of hair that he believed occurred only in Poland and that he attributed to the work of demons. The treatment he advised included purging by vomiting, emetics, and cleansing the blood. He also cited examples of "transplantation" or "transferral," in which a man could sometimes rid himself of illness by placing his excrement on a living plant. Such was mainstream medicine in the seventeenth century.[8]

Jewish students had to resist the temptation to lose their faith, for as Dr. Cohen warned, "No one (Jew) in all the lands of Italy, Poland, Germany and France should consider studying medicine without first filling his belly with the written and oral Torah and other subjects."[9]

In Poland there were entire families, father and son, grandson, and even great-grandson, of "Padua physicians," such as the DeLimas and Winklers in Posen, the DeJonases in Lemberg, the Marpurgos in Cracow, the Gordons in Vilna, and the Montaltos in Lublin. That they were respected by the populace is not surprising considering the number of unqualified practitioners extant.

As late as 1793, the Warsaw city records categorized Jewish physicians not by their diplomas or educational credentials but by the size and color of their beards, for example, "Dr. Salomon Hirszkowicz has a gray beard, Dr. Gerszon Baruchowicz has a sprouting beard, Dr. Felix Lieberman has a large beard . . ." and so on. Graduates of Padua may also have had beards, but unlike most of their colleagues they had academic degrees. Therefore, they were respected.[10]

According to David Ruderman, the Paduan experience was unique because for the first time a relatively large number of Jews graduated from a major medical school, entered the medical profession, and practiced across the entire European continent. It afforded the opportunity for intense socialization both among Jews from different backgrounds and non-Jewish students and faculty. As a result of a prolonged exposure to the liberal arts, classical texts, and the latest scientific advances, these impressionable youth were introduced to a new social network that endured after their graduation and constituted a significant cultural force. This emerging fraternity of intellectuals was nurtured by an enthusiasm and commitment to science and enlightenment along with a growing impatience for parochialism. Indeed, Ruderman suggests that the Paduan phenomenon represented a major vehicle for the diffusion of social culture in preemancipation Europe and served as a bridge for young Jewish intellectuals to the best of European civilization.[11]

8

Defensive Medicine

Among the many anti-Semitic acts promulgated during the time of Pope Pius IV (1555–1559), Christians were forbidden to employ Jewish physicians. With their livelihoods endangered, several individuals mounted a vigorous defense. Among these was David De Pomis (1525–1593), who in 1588 published a 127-page booklet, *De Medico Hebraeo Enarratio Apologia*, in response to the calumny contained in several papal bulls.[1]

De Pomis was born in Spoleto into a distinguished Jewish family that according to tradition was one of the four princely houses of Jerusalem carried off as captives by Titus to Rome in 70 C.E. He received his doctorate in medicine and philosophy in Perugia and then settled in Magliano near Rome, where he served both as physician and rabbi. He was granted permission to treat Christians by Pius IV, which was soon revoked by Pius V and later restored by Sixtus V.

In his *Apologia* De Pomis stressed that according to the Bible and Talmud, a Jewish physician must treat

every patient he encounters, and he cited famous examples, including such luminaries as Maimonides, Ibn
Ezra, and Gersonides. He declared that medicine was
discovered by the Jews long before the Greeks and later
revealed by them to the gentiles.

> Jewish physicians have been dwelling among the Chris-
> tians for 1,500 years. They have been regularly called
> to the sickbed of Christians; never as yet has anyone
> been charged with a crime. On the contrary they have
> distinguished themselves honorably among their pro-
> fessional colleagues. . . . No one has ever witnessed any
> crime by a Jewish physician and no one has received
> reliable information of such. It is only because of a
> common prejudice that we are accused and suffer in-
> jury. When Christians accept falsehood for truth, they
> harm themselves more than us, for this is completely
> contrary to the teachings of Christ. Why have princes
> and prelates sought Jewish physicians? Because of their
> crimes and wrongdoings or because of their ability and
> their good treatment?

Half a century after David De Pomis's scholarly
defense, another *Apologia* was published in Germany
by Benedict De Castro (1597–1684). He was the scion
of an illustrious family that included physicians in
Antwerp, Hamburg, Denmark, France, Holland, and
England. His father, Rodrigo De Castro (1546–1627), was
a famous physician and the author of a gynecology text.
Benedict received his early training from his father and
then continued his studies in Italy before returning to
his native Hamburg, where he was appointed president
of the Portuguese-Jewish community. For a time he was
physician to the queen of Sweden and flourished, but
late in life he was accused with others of forcibly con-

verting a Christian girl. He became impoverished and had to sell his books and furniture in order to survive.[2]

De Castro's *Apologia* was published in 1631 in response to an outpouring of slander directed against a small group of *converso* doctors who had found refuge in Hamburg. A pamphlet had been published anonymously that condemned "very famous men with a mass of falsehood and reproaches and in obscene manner." In his reply De Castro described the standard of ethical medical practice in these words:

> The true physician with his power over life and death, to whom the sick entrust themselves and all that they possess, must not rely on a beard, on splendid apparel, on arrogant appearance and a well-sounding name . . . [good physicians] not for the sake of honor or ambition but solely in the hope of improving human health, in relieving horrible epidemics, they combat the tyranny of disease with the salutary effects of medicinal plants and, with the placid hand of Aesculapius, they skillfully administer their remedies.

David De Pomis had lived freely as a Jew in Italy, but Benedict De Castro lived in a small community in Germany and had to be guarded in his talmudic citations. Nevertheless, he declared that "there is virtually no part of medicine that cannot be traced to the Hebrew forefathers," citing Solomon and Moses, "who laid the foundation of medicine as the most conspicuous of all arts," among others. About his Jewish medical colleagues he said, "They master several languages, which turns out to be a great advantage. Though scattered all over the world—as a matter of fact, they [Portuguese physicians] live in the north and among Christians—they manage to maintain the unity and purity of their nationality. I do not know what God wishes to do with and through them, but the one thing seems to be clear, that since the time when the world was created, no other nation has thus preserved its strength and integrity."

9

Portuguese Migrants

After the expulsion from Spain in 1492, many Jews fled to Portugal, but their acceptance was short-lived, and they soon spread out across Europe. In previous chapters I have described Portuguese *marrano* physicians who served the queens of France, Russia, Sweden, and England. Other *marranos* and New Christians gravitated to the relatively congenial Italian states or to Amsterdam and Turkey. A few traveled much farther to the distant East Indies or to the New World.

Abraham Zacutus Lusitanus (1575–1642) was a Portuguese *marrano* whose great-grandfather Abraham Zacutus (1452–1525) was a famous physician, astronomer, and historian. The younger Zacutus had a lucrative medical practice in Lisbon for thirty years, but in 1625 he was expelled and settled in Amsterdam. There he openly returned to Judaism, became circumcised, adopted the name Abraham, and began to write on medical subjects. His collected works, dedicated to King Louis XIII of France, were published in two huge volumes shortly after his death. They included a discussion of medical history, descriptions of diphtheria, blackwater fever, diseases of women, and a comprehensive spectrum of pathology and treatment. Of particular interest to the modern reader is his list of seventy-seven precepts, or rules of conduct, to be adhered to by a physician entering practice. They include the following:

- A physician shall be God-fearing.
- He shall be well dressed.
- He shall not indulge in unprofitable chatter.
- A physician shall not be miserly and niggardly.
- He shall not be primarily interested in fees.
- A physician shall have regard for the value of human life.
- He shall take a firm stance against popular prejudices.
- At times it is necessary to cheer up the patient with soft, kind words.
- In dispensing medicines, let him start with milder ones.
- Let him not treat every patient with medication; sometimes mere diet will do if the illness be mild and the patient weak.
- Let him always help nature, for that is the primary factor in health.
- If he cannot diagnose the case, let him be satisfied by merely prescribing a diet.
- He shall be careful in prescribing to the very young and the old, for they are weak.[1]

The decency and humility expressed in the above are reminiscent of the ideas expressed by Jewish physicians in earlier centuries (see chapter 3).

The voyages of Christopher Columbus and Vasco da Gama provided new opportunities for the wanderers to rebuild their shattered lives. Goa was established as the base of Portuguese operations in India in 1510, and many New Christians and *marranos* settled there. But no matter how far they roamed, the long arm of the Inquisition followed. Garcia de Orta, the son of New Christians, fled the Spanish Inquisition to Portugal and studied medicine, philosophy, and the arts at Salamanca. Later he became a professor of logic in Lisbon, but in 1534 he again felt obliged to flee, this time to the East Indies.

In Goa, de Orta's patients included governors and viceroys, one of whom granted him a lease on the island of Bombay, which at the time was only a small fishing village. There he maintained a botanical garden in which he grew medicinal herbs. He achieved fame as a naturalist and was the first European to describe several tropical diseases, notably Asiatic cholera. He led a protected life and never professed his Jewish origins. A year after his death, his sister was burned at the stake as "an impenitent Jewess," and in 1580, fourteen years after de Orta's death, his remains were exhumed and burned in an auto-da-fé as posthumous punishment for allegedly being a crypto-Jew during life.[2]

Spanish law forbade professing Jews from living in the New World's colonies, and medical practice was denied to anyone who was unable to prove four ancestral generations of Catholic blood. Auto-da-fés were held in Mexico and South America, where a number of Jewish physicians were killed during the sixteenth and seventeenth centuries.

With the British settlements to the north, the first recorded Jewish physician was Jacob Lumbruzo, who arrived from Lisbon in 1656. He developed a successful practice in Maryland and was known as "Ye Jew Doctor." Still, in 1658 he was tried for blasphemy, having become involved in a discussion on the doctrine of the Trinity. He escaped death only because of a general amnesty declared on the accession of Richard Cromwell. Another Portuguese, Samuel Nunez Ribiero, had attained eminence in his native Lisbon but was denounced to the Inquisition and imprisoned. His medical services were so needed that he was freed under the condition that two officers should reside with his family to guard against their relapsing into Judaism. He and his family escaped to England and from there set sail for Savannah, arriving in 1733, one year after the founding of Georgia. Dr. Ribiero was praised by Governor Oglethorpe, and the trustees of the colony gave him a land grant in gratitude for his medical services.[3]

Dr. John de Sequeyra (1712–1795) came from a London family of Portuguese Jewish origin that numbered many well-known physicians. In 1736 he left England to study medicine in Holland at the University of Leiden. His doctoral dissertation was dedicated to his brother, who practiced medicine in Goa. Why he chose to sail to Virginia in 1745 is not known—perhaps a spirit of adventure—but he settled in Williamsburg, where he practiced for fifty years.

Although de Sequeyra made no secret of his background, he did not visibly practice his religion. For twenty years he served as visiting physician for the Hospital for the Maintenance of Lunatics, Idiots, and Persons of Insane Mind, but he had to petition the Virginia Assembly for the fifty pounds a year that was owed to him.

During de Sequeyra's time a law established standard payment rates for physicians—five shillings for any visit in town or within five miles—with increments for longer distances and a double fee for those who had a university degree. The doctor attended Virginia's colonial governor, Lord Botecourt, who suffered from "bilious fever and Anthony's fire," and in 1769 he was called several times by Colonel George Washington to treat his stepdaughter, Martha Park Custis, who had epilepsy.

Dr. de Sequeyra was interested in horticulture, and in 1825 the president of William and Mary College wrote the following about him: "It is said by Mr. [Thomas] Jefferson that we are indebted to him for the introduction of the admirable vegetable the tomato. He was of the opinion that a person who should eat a sufficient abundance of these apples would never die. Whether he followed his own prescription is not known, but he certainly attained a very old age, and particularly for the climate in which he lived."[4]

Throughout the eighteenth century, increasing numbers of Jewish physicians from Germany and Holland traveled to the new lands. Records of the Spanish and Portuguese Synagogue in New York include Dr. Elias Woolin and a Dr. Nunez as early as 1742. During the War of 1812, Moses Sheftill and Jacob De la Motta were both army surgeons and later were among the founders of Savannah's congregation Mikve Israel. De la Motta gave the dedicatory address and contrasted the status of Jews in the United States with "their brethren in foreign lands, writhing under the shackles of odious persecution, and wild fanaticism. . . . On what spot in this habitable Globe does an Israelite enjoy more blessings, more privileges, or is more elevated in the sphere of preferment, and more conspicuously dignified in respectable stations?"[5]

Skipping ahead to the nineteenth century, one of America's outstanding clinical teachers was Jacob Mendez Da Costa (1833–1900), who was so well respected that he was called "the physician's physician." His family had emigrated from Portugal to England in the sixteenth century, but he was born on the island of St. Thomas. He graduated from Jefferson Medical College in Philadelphia in 1852 at the age of nineteen and studied there and later in Europe with some of the most famous physicians of the nineteenth century, including Meigs, Pancoast, Bernard, Broca, Trousseau, and Rokitansky. During his career, he won many honorary degrees and awards. His book *Medical Diagnosis* appeared in nine editions during his lifetime, and he was immortalized for generations of medical students by the syndrome that still bears his name. Da Costa's syndrome (1871) or "irritable heart," later known also as "soldier's heart" or neurocirculatory asthenia, was appreciated by him to be a common cause of disability among the soldiers he cared for during the Civil War and which he concluded was due to psychological stress rather than physical disease.[6]

From these biographical sketches it is clear that the Sephardic Jewish medical influence was felt throughout the world for centuries after the expulsions from Spain and Portugal.

10

Eighteenth-Century
Medical Vignettes

During the eighteenth century there were fewer than three hundred trained physicians in the entire Russian Empire, and so it is no surprise that for the vast majority of the general population who lived in the countryside, or in the case of most of the Jews in small towns and villages, medical care was supervised by a mélange of healers, midwives, bloodletters, bonesetters, masseurs, sorcerers, and soothsayers. The common people of Russia and Poland were more likely to get their advice from barbers, bathhouse attendants, and wise old women than from doctors. Many Jews relied upon amulets and incantations to ward off the evil eye, although most rabbis condemned their use.[1]

In truth, there was little that distinguished medical care among the Jews from that of their gentile neighbors—cupping, bleeding, and leeching were normal, and folk remedies were sometimes bizarre or even grotesque. During this medically undisciplined period, when medical information was provided by people of dubious qualifications, the few trained physicians stressed adherence to basic principles of hygiene that was consistent with biblical and rabbinic teaching. The following narratives provide a general sense of the time:

An amusing insight into what can befall the amateur dabbler appeared in the autobiography of Solomon Maimon (1754–1800), a brilliant if erratic philosopher who was one of the first Poles to fall under the influence of the German Jewish Enlightenment. As a young *yeshivah* student in Lithuania, the young Salomon ben Joshua was sufficiently influenced by Maimonides' writings that he adopted the family name of Maimon. Evidently, he studied Maimonides' works so carefully that he believed he was accomplished enough to practice medicine. His own words describe what happened:

> From my generous friend the chief rabbi, I received two medical books . . . in connection with every disease is given an explanation of its cause, its symptoms, and the method of its cure, along with even the ordinary prescription for their cure. But in this practice things turned out very comically. If a patient told me some of his symptoms, I guessed from them the nature of the disease itself and inferred the presence of the other symptoms. If the patient said that he had none of these, I stubbornly insisted on their being present all the same. . . . Prescriptions I could never keep in my head, so that when I prescribed anything, I was obliged to go home first and look it up. How this succeeded may be imagined. It had at least this good result, that I saw something more was surely required for a practical physician than I understood at the time.[2]

Such a "practical" physician was Dr. Abraham Wolf, who in 1756 published a treatise for Polish people about preventing cholera, which advised that "the rooms must be frequently heated, the windows opened, cleanliness observed, dairy food eaten, alcohol avoided, and water imbibed with vinegar or Rhine wine. One should take hot baths and perspire excessively, and avoid anger, fear, and grief, which have a debilitating effect on the body"— all sound principles. Dr. Wolf also praised the efficacy of almond oil, camphor, tobacco, and a potion made of lilacs, honey, and vinegar to be drunk every quarter of an hour.[3]

Another product of the German Enlightenment was Dr. Moshe Marcuse, who moved from Koenigsberg to Poland in 1773 and later settled in a *shtetl* in the Ukraine. In order to reach the populace, he published a book in Yiddish, *Sefer Refu'ot* (*Book of Cures*), which described the economic hardships of the Jews, their cultural backwardness, and their unsanitary living conditions. For those for whom no doctor was available, he transmitted elementary medical knowledge and emphasized proper nourishment and cleanliness. He exhorted the masses to use only qualified physicians and advised Jewish communities to "examine the diplomas of practicing physicians and investigate their education to determine whether they possess the right to practice medicine."[4]

A different kind of professional advice was given by Isaac Erter (1791–1851), who was born in the Galician city of Brody and began to study medicine in Budapest at age thirty-three. Erter wrote, "I am a physician and my profession is to heal wounds and to find remedies for curing disease. Though learned physicians with high-sounding titles think themselves superior to me and look down upon me, I nevertheless cure as well as they do and my dead revive as little as do theirs."

Dr. Erter was a scathing satirist, and among his targets were those physicians who abused their profession either out of ignorance or the pursuit of wealth and fame. His wit still has a bite that is evident from the following "golden aphorisms" by observance of which Erter claimed "even a medical ass will fill his treasury with gold":

1. Powder your hair white and keep on the table of your study a human skull and some animal skeletons. Those coming to you for medical advice will then think that your hair has turned white through constant study and overwork in your profession.

2. Fill your library with large books, richly bound in red and gold. Though you never even open them, people will be impressed with your wisdom.

3. Sell or pawn everything, if that is necessary, to have a carriage of your own.

4. When called to a patient, pay less attention to him than to those about him. On leaving the sickroom assume a grave face and pronounce the case a most critical one. Should the patient die, you will be understood to have hinted at his death; if, on the other hand, he recovers, his relations and friends will naturally attribute his recovery to your skill.

5. Have as little as possible to do with the poor, as they will only send for you in hopeless and desperate cases; you will gain neither honor nor reward by attending them. Let them wait outside your house, that passersby may be amazed at the crowd patiently waiting to obtain your services.

6. Consider every medical practitioner as your natural enemy and speak of him always with the utmost disparagement. If he is a student of history dabbling in the annals of the past, say his work is alien to the practice of medicine. If he be young, you must say he has not had suffi-

cient experience; if he be old, you must declare that his
eyesight is bad, or that he is more or less crazy, and not
to be trusted in important cases.[5]

An extreme example of professional competition
that played out in London between medical leaders
respectively of the Ashkenazic and Sephardic communities provides insight into Jewish social dynamics of
the eighteenth century. There was animosity between
the Ashkenazim and the larger and more affluent Sephardim. The Royal College of Physicians was the preeminent medical organization, and no physician could practice in the London area unless he was a licentiate and
had been approved by the Censor's Board. Admission
generally was restricted to graduates of Oxford and
Cambridge universities. Notwithstanding, there also were
a "bold and ignorant multitude of empirics" practicing
in London including, according to one critic, "former
tinkers, toothdrawers, pedlars, porters, horse-gelders,
horse-leeches, idiots, apple-squires, broomsmen, bawds,
witches, conjurers, sow gelders, rogues, rat-catchers,
renegades, and proctors of spittle houses."[6]

Dr. Meyer Low Schomberg (1690–1761), a Jewish
immigrant from Germany, arrived in London in 1720.
He was of a quarrelsome nature but was an able physician and built a large practice. A footnote in Boswell's
The Life of Samuel Johnson (1791) states, "Fothergill, a
Quaker, and Schomberg, a Jew, had the greatest practice of physicians of their time." Schomberg was elected
a Fellow of the Royal College of Physicians in 1726. One
of his chief professional rivals was Sephardic physician
Jacob de Castro Sarmento, a Portuguese who fled the
Inquisition and came to England in 1720. Sarmento was
the author of two medical books and helped to popu-

larize the use of cinchona, but when he was proposed for fellowship in the Royal College, Schomberg wrote a letter that repeated a previously discredited calumny that Sarmento had been guilty of betraying some of his brethren to the Inquisitor. Nevertheless Sarmento was elected to the college.

The acrimony continued when Schomberg spread a rumor that "Sarmento was an ass and a fool" because he had used an improper dose of an opiate in treating a prominent member of the Sephardic community. Sarmento reported the matter to the Censor's Board of the college, who agreed and fined Dr. Schomberg four pounds. Meyer Schomberg never forgave the college for this humiliation, and a running battle continued that even involved the medical careers of his twin sons, who followed in their father's footsteps. The messy affair was recently detailed by Alex Sakul, who described it as "the notorious Schomberg *shemozzle*."[7]

11

Who Really Wrote "Maimonides' Prayer"?

The authenticity of the Physician's Prayer, which traditionally was attributed to Maimonides, has been debated since early in this century. Sir William Osler wrote to Dr. Joseph Hertz (1872–1946), the chief rabbi of Great Britain, for an opinion and after due investigation, Dr. Hertz replied: "The Prayer is the product of Dr. Markus Herz [apparently no relation], a friend and pupil of Immanuel Kant and Moses Mendelssohn. He was a physician in the Jewish Hospital in Berlin. The Prayer was composed by him in the German language [in 1783]. . . . The current English version seems to be from the Hebrew translation and first appeared in the London paper *Voice of Jacob* on the 24th of December, 1841."[1]

Who was Markus Herz? To be mentioned in the same context as Maimonides, he must have been a man of great intellect and sensitivity. The following is extracted from a biographical study by Brigitte Ibing:

Herz was born in 1747 in Berlin at a time when the Jewish population was living in the city illegally. His father was an impoverished Torah scribe who provided the young man with a *yeshivah* education. At age fifteen, he moved to Koenigsberg with the intention of becoming a merchant. He had the good fortune to befriend the prosperous and highly cultivated Friedlander family and became a protege of Joachim Moses Friedlander. The youth attended Kant's lectures and began to study medicine, which was the only field of higher study then open to Jews. His studies in philosophy led him to the idea that natural and humanistic sciences should be integrated and he urged that subjects like zoology and botany should be limited in favor of what today would be called psychology or psychosomatic medicine. He found it to be unsatisfactory that the universities were able to find professors who knew every bone and ligament, but not one who could teach medical psychology.[2]

Herz strove to introduce understanding of the patient's psyche into his own medical practice in Berlin, where he worked from 1774 until his death at age fifty-six in 1803. He became successful and often visited up to thirty patients a day, mostly on foot, and treated patients regardless of their social class. In addition to private practice, along with his father-in-law he headed the Jewish Hospital (*hekdesh*), and under their humane leadership the hospital developed an excellent reputation for, among other things, its cleanliness, a rare quality in those times. Although himself not religiously observant, he arranged for strict Jewish dietary and ceremonial laws.

Herz was a leader of Berlin's Jewish Enlightenment, and beginning in 1776 he and his beautiful and brilliant young wife, Henrietta, held lectures in their home concerning medical science, physics, philosophy, and logic.[3]

In his audience were leading intellectuals and members of the royal house, including the crown prince. The same prince became Friedrich Wilhelm II, who in 1787 appointed Herz as the first Jewish professor of medicine in Prussia. There may be some traditionalists who still maintain that Maimonides composed the Physician's Prayer, but whether Markus Herz composed it or merely translated an earlier prayer from Hebrew into German, he surely was an impressive and worthy figure in his own right who strove to introduce spirituality and psychology into medical theory and practice.

12

The Late Entry
of Russian Physicians

When Polish and Russian students began to receive
their medical education in western Europe, an important by-product of their travels was that they were
exposed to and many became advocates of the Jewish
Enlightenment (*haskalah*), which helped to introduce
secular thinking into their intellectually stagnant Jewish communities. Therefore, it is no surprise that on their
return home these first trained Jewish physicians were
not greeted with unbridled enthusiasm. Indeed, they
often were perceived as competition by the wonderworkers, folk healers, and hasidic rebbes whom the
doctors regarded as charlatans. The founder of Hasidism,
known by the initials BeShT for Baal Shem Tov, who
was born about 1698, in his early years was a common
healer who made use of plants and herbs, bloodletting,
charms, and even ground-up diamonds.[1]

Even before the advent of the hasidic movement,
kabbalists such as Rabbi Joel Baal Shem made use of
amulets, special remedies, and incantations. Although

not certified physicians, they brought light and hope to ignorant masses. Since these healers performed magic cures using the Name of God, they were called "Baal Shem," master of the Name of God. Some prescribed parts of nonkosher animals (snake, fox, raven, even pig), having borrowed these remedies from gentile folk medical practice, and they were particularly sought after to cure mental disorders or to exorcise demons. To give them their due, their advice often was based on sound hygienic and dietary principles: do not sleep more than eight hours and not less than six; upon arising in the morning, fling your extremities around (exercise); every week skip one meal; moderation in everything, particularly in food, drink, and sex.[2]

Rabbi Jacob Emden, in his writings on medicine, was skeptical of the profession's claim to a superior understanding of health and illness and was unwilling to accept the testimony of physicians in declaring a patient's illness life threatening. The degree of certainty of professional medical knowledge was too low to serve as a basis for violating Jewish law in order to save a life.[3]

Some maintained that medicine had regressed compared to earlier times. Rabbi Jonathan Eybeschuetz (1690–1764) said, "You should not take notice of the later doctors . . . they have become foolish and stupid in their knowledge . . . they understand nature as little as a dog that licks the sea." On the other hand, Rabbi Saul Berlin, also writing in the late eighteenth century, ruled that one may violate the Sabbath to fulfill medical instructions, even those issued by a non-Jew. Rabbi Nahman of Bratzlav (d. 1811), the great-grandson of the Baal Shem Tov, urged his followers to resort to prayers of the *tzaddik* rather than to use medicines.[4]

Dr. Baruch Ben Jacob Schick (1740?–1812), some-times known as Baruch Shklover after his native city, was ordained as a rabbi in 1764, but although he usually is referred to as a physician, there is doubt whether he ever had a formal medical education; more likely, he was self-taught. Nevertheless, he achieved a reputation and late in life served as court physician to Prince Radziwill in the Polish city of Slutzk. He was influenced by a meet-ing with the Vilna Gaon, who advised him to translate scientific works into Hebrew as a way of attaining a bet-ter understanding of Torah. The Gaon recognized a basic linkage between knowledge of religion and of science, and as a result of this encounter Schick translated Euclid's book on geometry, *The Elements*, into Hebrew. Dr. Schick viewed science as having "flowed from the fountain of Judah," and wishing to restore Jewish science to its origi-nal status, passionately encouraged his people to rouse themselves from their ignorance. Schick also studied as-tronomy, languages, mathematics, and philosophy and was an important transitional figure who served as a bridge between the rabbi-scholar physicians of earlier times and the secular scientists who would emerge in the next century.[5, 6]

Jewish students in those parts of Poland under Austro–Hungarian sovereignty were permitted to enter medical schools as early as 1782, as a result of Emperor Joseph II's Act of Tolerance, and the first class of the medical-surgical academy in Warsaw included a Jew, Jakub Novak, among its twenty-seven graduates.[7] How-ever, in Russia the youth of the world's largest Jewish community still had to go abroad to pursue their medi-cal studies, and those who returned had to pass special examinations in order to obtain a license. It was not until reforms initiated by Alexander II in the 1860s brought unprecedented opportunities that there was a surge of young Russian Jews, as well as other minorities, even serfs, into medical schools. In 1865 Jewish physicians were granted the right to enter government service as well as the right of unrestricted residence throughout Russia, and in 1879 these rights were extended to Jewish feldshers (see chapter 13).

A few multitalented physician-scholars continued to operate within a religious framework. One such was Hayyim David Bernard (1782–1858), born near Piotrkow, who at the age of fourteen traveled to Berlin to study medicine. The liberal policies of King Frederick William II enabled him to become a court physician and later a medical officer in the Prussian army—a considerable achievement for a Jew. After Napoleon's conquest of Poland, Dr. Bernard was appointed medical inspector for the Warsaw region. A typical product of the German Jewish Enlightenment, at first he remained aloof from Polish Jewry, but a spiritual crisis led him to approach Rabbi Jacob Horowitz, the Seer of Lublin. Bernard became strictly Orthodox and a follower of the Seer. He grew a beard but continued to wear Western clothes and never mastered Yiddish. He became a leading communal figure venerated by Jews and Christians alike and spent the rest of his life as head of the hospital in Piotrkow and as a wonder-working *hasid*. For decades after his death, Dr. Bernard's grave was a center of hasidic pilgrimage.[8]

Another example of a pious Jewish physician was Dr. Ephraim Edelstein (1803–1883) who, after being ordained as a rabbi, went to Vienna to study medicine and then returned to Lomza, Poland, to serve as chief physician of the local Jewish hospital. He made a point of conversing only in Yiddish but also was a Polish patriot and, during the uprising against Russia in 1863, organized a clandestine field hospital to care for wounded Polish fighters.[9]

To many observant Jews, the new breed of physicians was seen as acculturated destroyers of the tradition, and their credibility was questioned because of their doubtful level of religious observance. It was as if having eaten the forbidden fruit of modern science, they were tainted and had forfeited their role as proper intermediaries between man and God. In the 1840s, when the renowned Rabbi Israel Salanter learned that his son had gone to Berlin to study medicine, he removed his shoes and observed *shivah*, seven days of mourning.[10]

Conditions in the medical schools were harsh and a medical career was considered beneath the dignity of the sons of the privileged classes. One historian observed that those who pursued a medical career came "from those segments of society not distinguished by gentleness of habit or by cultivation." Physicians were classified as artisans of the same low social status as porters and piano tuners. Nonetheless, for the underprivileged a medical career was an opportunity for upward social mobility and for some Jewish physicians served as a passport out of the restricted areas.[11]

Times were changing rapidly, and by the 1860s many believed that becoming "Russified" and participating in the mainstream culture was like "starving persons suddenly treated to a delicious meal." The ambition of many of the wealthy no longer was to have a son-in-law who was well versed in Torah but, instead, a graduate from a university, the possessor of a diploma. In the Jewish ethos, wisdom was a fundamental value and in this increasingly

secularized age, the social distinction of having an educated son in a respected profession equaled or exceeded
financial or religious considerations.

Among the prominent Jewish physician-scholars of
this period was Judah Leib Benjamin Katzenelson (1846–
1917). Born in Chernigov, Ukraine, he studied at the
yeshivot of Bobruisk in ByeloRussia, but he became
attracted to the *haskalah* and believed that its empha-
sis on trades and agriculture would solve the problems
of Russian Jewry. He studied medicine at the Military
Medical Academy of St. Petersburg, where he subsequently practiced. He also was a journalist and historian and published a number of studies about medical
disorders as described in the Torah and Talmud.[12]

Dr. Isaac Kaminer (1834–1901) was another Jewish physician who was smitten by the secular world.
Born in a small Ukrainian town near Zhitomir, Kaminer
studied under a Hebrew teacher his parents engaged
to instruct him in the usual exclusively religious education. He had a quick mind, and it was hoped that the
boy would become a rabbi. When he showed signs of
straying from the rigid path prescribed for him, his parents arranged for an early marriage, but the responsibilities of a burgeoning family failed to deter him. In
1857 he gave up his position as a teacher in a rabbinical seminary, left his wife and five children, and entered
the university in Kiev. He was adept in mathematics and
physics but realized that as a Jew the only way to support his family was through a medical career. Kaminer
struggled through and eventually became a prominent
physician who traveled from village to village to visit
the sick. Somehow he found the time to become a poet
and essayist and in his writings spoke out against social

injustice. He became attracted to socialism and later became an enthusiastic Zionist.[13]

After the assassination of the relatively liberal Czar Alexander II in 1881, harsh discriminatory laws were enacted that again denied government positions to Jewish doctors. In 1887 the imperial government established quotas for Jewish students in all institutions of higher learning; in St. Petersburg no more than 3 percent of a medical school class could be Jewish, compared to about 10 percent a decade before. Those who were able to overcome the restrictions gravitated toward private practice and neglected fields that were less attractive to their gentile colleagues, such as dermatology–venereology or what was called "microscopy," a hybrid of hematology, histology, and pathology.

Zionism was among the emerging political causes of this period, and many Jewish physicians, including Max Mandelstamm (1839–1912), were among its advocates. Mandelstamm was born in Lithuania to enlightened parents who sent him to a Russian high school. He entered medical school in Estonia but transferred to Kharkov University and later studied ophthalmology in Germany. He became a prominent specialist and opened an eye clinic in Kiev, where he joined the medical faculty. Three times his colleagues elected him to the rank of associate professor, but each time he was rejected by the university council because of his religion. The pogroms of 1881 inspired him to become a Zionist and, in time, he became a close friend and associate of Theodor Herzl.[14]

As in earlier times, some Jewish physicians achieved fame in nonmedical fields. Leo Pinsker (1821–1912) of Odessa, an internist who was decorated by the czar for his excellent volunteer work in the Russian army during the Crimean War, was one of the founders of Zionism. Notable among the intellectual elite were the poet Saul Tchernichovsky (1875–1943)[15] and ophthalmologist Ludwig Zamenhof (1859–1917), the creator of the universal language Esperanto.

13

"My Son the Feldsher"

Until this century, because there were so few trained physicians in rural areas or in small towns in eastern Europe, an important underclass of health practitioners were the feldshers. Their antecedents were medieval barber-surgeons who were recruited into the German and Swiss armies as mercenaries. The original German word *feldscherer* literally meant a military man working with shears. The tradition of bloodletting by barbers dated back to 1215, when the Christian Church, disturbed about the excess letting of blood by monks, prohibited the clergy from practicing surgery altogether. By default the technique was assumed by barbers, and in sixteenth-century Europe to be a barber was to have a foot on the lowest rung of the medical ladder; in addition to cutting hair, curling wigs, and shaving whiskers, a barber might pull teeth, dress wounds, and do at first minor, then major, surgery. Indeed, the father of modern surgery, Ambroise Pare (born c. 1510), began as a barber-surgeon.[1]

This phenomenon began in western Europe but spread rapidly to the east, where feldshers became particularly numerous. Some of them were well educated and relatively accomplished. For example, Issachar bar Teller, a Jewish barber-surgeon, practiced in seventeenth-century Prague and claimed that his "master and teacher" was the esteemed physician Joseph Shelomoh Delmedigo. Teller published a small medical self-help book for laymen in which he gave advice in Yiddish, but he warned his readers to seek medical help in the case of serious disease. Unlike many practitioners of his time, he was skeptical of the value of astrology and noted that excessive bloodletting was potentially dangerous: "We Jews use bloodletting without rhyme or reason; this I can observe every day, but I am powerless to prevent it."[2]

Russian feldshers at first had only practical experience, but by the early nineteenth century professional schools were established. Initially, the curricula of these schools were limited, but by the late nineteenth century the course for feldshers was extended to four years.[3,4] Increasing numbers of Jewish youth became feldshers, and although their relative proportions to physicians varied according to location and changing government regulations, in 1887 in the Pale of Settlement feldshers outnumbered physicians 817 to 480 and in the kingdom of Poland feldshers outnumbered physicians 1,051 to 198. While Jews constituted only about 4 percent of the entire population, they comprised 28 percent of the total number of feldshers versus just over 6 percent of all Russian doctors. By the end of the nineteenth century, almost all towns with a Jewish population of twenty thousand or more had Jewish hospitals with at least one Jewish physician and a few feldshers and midwives.

Although the smaller communities did not have a resident physician, practically all had feldshers who, if they were licensed, displayed the official insignia of three copper plates on a rod derived from the barber's basin.

Some feldshers were relatively well-to-do and, because they remained religiously observant members of the community, they were popular with the masses. This was in contrast with the generally assimilated physicians, most of whom rarely were seen in synagogue or at Jewish gatherings, smoked and rode in public on Saturdays, and eschewed Yiddish for Polish or Russian. Furthermore, since few people could afford the physician's fees, they generally were called only as a last resort and the outcomes of their treatments probably were little better than that of their competitors. Late in the nineteenth century, Jewish physicians again were denied government positions, which forced them to make a living through fee-for-service private practice, further exacerbating professional competition with the feldshers. The profession of feldsher was abolished by the new Polish government after the end of World War I.

In fact, most people were more interested in results than in medical degrees, and distinctions between the different categories of practitioners sometimes were ambiguous, particularly in rural areas. The traditional Jewish term for healer, *rofe* in Hebrew, *roife* in Yiddish, didn't have an academic connotation, and the generic term *doktor* was used indiscriminately. Technically, the feldsher was a physician's assistant and did cupping, leeching, and performed other procedures that were considered below the trained doctor's dignity. However, many so-called *rofes* in reality were feldshers.

Regardless of their background, these unschooled healers relied on empiric observation, and they often were the laughingstock of the more intelligent classes, who would exaggerate their ignorance. This is exemplified by the story of a cobbler who took sick. The healer was called, diagnosed a severe case of typhoid, and muttered to himself, "There's no hope." Overhearing these words, the cobbler feebly prayed to be given one last enjoyment before dying. To his taste nothing was sweeter or more palatable than sauerkraut. Could he have a last dish? The healer agreed; the cobbler had his fill of sauerkraut and miraculously recovered. On hearing this, the healer was overjoyed and wrote in his prescription book, "A tested cure for advanced typhoid is sauerkraut." Soon afterward, the same healer was called to the bed of another patient, this time a tailor. The diagnosis again was severe typhoid. Of course sauerkraut was prescribed, but the next day the tailor was dead. Unperturbed, the healer wrote in his prescription book, "Sauerkraut effective only under the condition that the patient is a cobbler. It will not work in case he happens to be a tailor."[5] Now that's empiric medicine!

On a personal note, I have a patient named Joseph Felcher, who was born in Poland. He doesn't know of any physicians in his family tree, but he recalls how as a child his sleep often was disturbed by loud banging on the apartment door and calls for "Feldsher." Someone had a toothache or another ailment. My patient has an elderly Russian uncle who when drafted into the army was assigned to the medical unit only because of his name. He was afraid to admit that he had no medical experience and risk being sent to the front. He had a meteoric career, eventually became head of an army hospital, and was personally decorated by Joseph Stalin.

14

Shtetl Medicine

The following account from Chaim Aronson's (1825–1888) autobiography depicts life in a small Lithuanian *shtetl* and what happened when as a child he contracted a high fever:

In those days there was no quinine available in the small towns, nor were there physicians; the only healers were the quacks, every one of whom was a charlatan. There were also the old women who knew every remedy in the world, including those of the miracle workers and the Tartars and the magicians, and they offered their advice and treatment to all the sick. I did not escape their attentions.

The first remedy my father tried on me was one prescribed by the Rabbi: he had to write over all the doors and windows of the house and to chalk upon all the walls in large letters "The boy Hayyim is not at home." The idea was that when the demon of malaria came to visit me, he would see written everywhere that the boy he was seeking was not home, and therefore would turn away and go back to wherever he came from. Unfortunately, the demon of malaria did not read Yiddish, and so he paid me constant visits.[1]

When home remedies failed, a call might go out to the local "enema woman." Since the cause of illness was presumed to be something that had gotten in, it had to be eliminated, and the enema woman was a dread figure to the children of many a *shtetl*. Devoting herself exclusively to this arcane art, her apparatus in its most primitive form was a calf's bladder and a goose quill, and her treatment was threatened as a cure for any ailment, including naughtiness.

The next level of health care required the services of the healer (*rofe*), who in some locales was a feldsher. One could communicate with him in simple Yiddish, and the family and neighbors and the sick person himself took an active part in the proceedings, even giving their own opinions and advice. The friendly healer listened patiently without offending anyone. He would administer leeches, dry and wet cupping glasses (*bankes*), bloodletting, and might examine the patient with a stethoscope just like a physician. It was for him to say whether a doctor should be consulted, and if one was called, whether his prescriptions should be followed. Memorial books of the various communities often recalled the healers with affection. The following account describes Shloyme, the Healer of Bilgoray:

> Three brass plates hung by the healer's door, the symbol of his craft [in fact, the symbol of the feldsher]. Actually he hadn't finished his degree; he had served as a medic in the Russian army and when his tour of duty was over, he became the town healer. He wore a

stiff black top hat and a pointed little beard and he was the only man in town who wore a short jacket. He used to wash with perfumed soap, and it was whispered among the women that the healer ate tomatoes, which were held to be nonkosher at that time. When he made a house call he was received with great honor and the family hung on his every word. He asked the invalid to describe his pain, checked his pulse and took out various instruments from the little bag he carried with him. He checked the patient's throat and then gave him aspirin. . . . In addition, he applied cups and leeches, painted throats, and gave enemas. Anyone who had a toothache went to Shloyme the Healer. Shloyme would sit him down on his chair, grab hold of the tooth, and before the patient could scream, Shloyme handed the tooth back to him.[2]

Only when the healer became alarmed was the trained physician called in as a specialist consultant, but unless the patient was near death or very wealthy, the waiting list to see him was long. The highest accolade for a prosperous physician was the title "professor," which was more a mark of general distinction than of academic rank. The following story illustrates the special status afforded the physician:

In extreme cases, with both reluctance and fear, the doctor is called . . . a figure of awe, waited on hand and foot and deferred to by everyone. He sits in state while the family stands around him, the women craning and staring. His instruments, his learning, his foreign appearance and manner inspire wonder and uneasiness. Everyone competes to bring him whatever he asks for— a spoon, some water, a towel—and to fetch his coat when he is ready to leave. As he goes, the father tim-

idly shakes hands with him and shyly presses the fee
into his palm.[3]

East European Jewish folklore was full of superstition and belief in magic was part of the popular culture
of *shtetl* life. There was no specific prohibition against
consulting a magician, even a non-Jewish magician, to
seek a cure. Although rationalists denounced the use
of magic and amulets, their admonitions had little influence, and in one form or another superstitious practices persisted and continue to persist in some places
even to the present time.

If one listens to east European Jews conversing,
their speech often is sprinkled with *kaynahoras*, the
contraction of the Yiddish *Keyen ayen hore*, meaning
"May there be no evil eye."

Q: "How are you?"
A: "*Kaynahora*, not bad."

Tradition holds that trouble can be averted merely
by saying the word—the kind of trouble that arises from
jealousy of good fortune, be it health, wealth, beauty,
or some other desirable quality. The evil eye was perceived as a free-floating malevolence that attacked those
who were most vulnerable and most favored—the young,
the talented, the attractive.[4]

Avoiding the evil eye included avoiding any expres-
sion of happiness or of praise, or at least qualifying any
such statement. The answer to the salutation "How are
you?" was not "Fine" but "Not bad" or some other less-
than-enthusiastic affirmative. A child might be covered
with a dirty bag or given an ugly name because beauty
should be veiled. A costly garment should not be spread

over the bed when guests visit lest it "burn the eye of the guests," and precious glass should be broken at a wedding. Similarly, amulets in the shape of an outstretched hand and containing a holy verse or a protective red band tied around the wrist or neck of a newborn child were used to avert the evil eye.

Fear of the evil eye was not uniquely Jewish. Indeed, the belief was prevalent in Babylonian, Egyptian, and Persian texts and later in Christian culture. Judaism generally gave less credence to magic and superstition than others, but in ancient and early medieval times, the rabbis had to deal with the seeming reality of the evil eye on a daily basis. In the Talmud, for example, two leading rabbinic authorities, Abaye and Raba, often were in heated opposition to each other but agreed that "nothing done for purposes of healing is to be forbidden as superstitious." In only one respect did Jewish folk medicine differ substantially from its gentile counterpart in that ingestion of blood was abhorrent and there are no known instances of the prescription of blood for internal use (Babylonian Talmud, *Shabbat* 67a and *Hullin* 77b).

The idea that some eyes have the power to harm at a glance was an accepted phenomenon in early midrashic literature. Sarah cast the evil eye on Hagar (*Genesis Rabbah* 45:4), Joseph's brothers on Joseph (*Genesis Rabbah* 84:10), the evil eye caused the breaking of the first tablets of the law (*Numbers Rabbah* 12:4), and so on. One talmudic rabbi stated that "ninety-nine persons die from the evil eye and only one dies a natural death"—a formidable statistic.

Joseph's name often was invoked because he was the prototype of the individual who conquered the evil eye and always was his own person. A contemporary

rabbi, Shlomo Riskin, cites his mentor Rav J. B. Solo-
veitchik's explanation that the evil eye refers to an individual who watches how others look at him and endeavors only to act in a manner that will please *them*.
Playing to the eyes of others instead of dancing to the
tune of God, therefore, is understood to be evil and
destructive.[5]

A different moral lesson is that all people should
take care against looking enviously at their neighbor's
possessions. One commentator has listed over eighty
anti-evil eye practices among east European Jews, and
a two-volume book on the subject written in 1910 was
considered by its author as the "inadequate work of a
beginner." Later he published two more volumes.

In addition to the evil eye, there were many other
superstitious beliefs related to health. The following
compendium selected from Joshua Trachtenberg's *Jewish Magic and Superstition* only begins to scratch the
surface:

- Frightening a person may scare the invading spirit out—
  for example, frightening away hiccups.
- What tastes vile to the patient also is vile to the demon—thus the medicinal value of items such as skull,
  marrow, fat, sweat, semen. Rubbing warm urine over
  a gouty joint was basic medicine.
- Cobwebs rubbed into an open wound stop the bleeding.
- Encircling an abscess or rash or sore spot with the finger or with some object such as a ring while reciting a
  charm bans the evil spirit from working within the con-
  fined area.
- An illness can be transferred to an animal, or to an in-
  animate object, or to someone else. The story was told
  that once a man was mortally ill and another jokingly

said to him, "I'll buy your illness from you for such and such a sum." The invalid promptly responded, "It's a bargain." Immediately, he arose cured and the purchaser sickened and died.

- Evil demons could be outwitted by prayer, giving charity, changing conduct, or changing name. It was as if the one who changed his name said to the demon, "I am not the person you are seeking" and was taken at his word. Hoodwinking angels and demons was commonplace when an illness was prolonged and severe. The new name usually suggested a long, healthy life such as Hayim ("life"), Alter ("old man"), or Zeide ("grandfather").[6]

Likewise, the stories of Isaac Bashevis Singer contain a particularly loathsome pharmacopoeia of folk medicines that were prevalent in the *shtetls* of Poland. The following are only a few:

roasted garlic and salted peas to restore sexual potency.
moldy preserves to dispel sadness.
finger and toenails kneaded into a lump and thrown to a dog to cure epilepsy.
a stew made of foreskin of newly circumcised boy, virgin blood of a bride, devil's dung, fried frogs, placenta of a newborn child, and stag's testicles to induce pregnancy.[7]

Where did they obtain the ingredients? Today we take perverse delight in recalling the noisome and naive folk remedies of yesteryear. Certainly they were not exclusively a Jewish phenomenon. The idea was that the more odious, the more potent; if offensive to the patient, even more so to the invader.

As Jews emerged from their isolated *shtetl* lives, they retained many of their popular old beliefs, but gradually as they entered the mainstream they began to accommodate modern medical approaches.

15

The Lower East Side

The first Jewish doctors to come to America had been Sephardic but during the 1860s to 1880s were predominantly German. At midcentury, New York City had some ten thousand to twelve thousand mostly German-Jews out of a total population of a half million. A cholera epidemic in 1849 galvanized the community into establishing the Jews' Hospital (later Mount Sinai Hospital), which was founded in 1852 and began exclusively accepting Jewish patients in 1855.[1]

One of the Jews' Hospital's first attending physicians was Abraham Jacobi (1830–1919), who in the manner of European students of the day had studied medicine in several German universities before graduating from Bonn in 1851. He ran into difficulties with the authorities for alleged revolutionary activities, was imprisoned, escaped to England, and came to America in 1853. In his first year of practice Jacobi earned 973 dollars by charging 25 cents for office visits, 50 cents for house calls, and 5 to 10 dollars for obstetrical cases. For a while he provided consultations from behind the prescription counter of a local drugstore, keeping 25 cents for himself and paying 25 cents to the pharmacist.

Dr. Jacobi was a prolific writer, teacher, historian, and lecturer and became a scholar of international reputation, generally credited as being "the father of the specialty of pediatrics." An early advocate of breast-feeding and possibly the first to appreciate the significance of boiling milk (1877), he introduced bedside teaching in the United States, held the first academic chair as professor of pediatrics in the country, founded the American Pediatrics Society, and in 1912 was elected president of the American Medical Association.[2, 3, 4]

In 1905, Dr. Jacobi addressed the graduates of the Washington University medical department in St. Louis, and this extract gives an amusing insight into medical practice of the day, with which the modern physician can empathize:

Exercise and rest, open windows, hygiene in general, diet in particular, hot and cold water are together a panacea when judiciously ordered. Frequently you may do without the apothecary. Then, however, your patient may turn upon you.

"Exercise, open windows, starving, cold water, no tobacco, no coffee, no highball, and no prescription? Doctor, is that all? I know that much myself. I see that I must go somewhere else. Now doctor, really, is there any bill?"

He does not appreciate that you have given him the quintessence of two thousand years worth of medicine, goes to your neighbor, who gives him no quintessences, no two thousand years worth of study, but a prescription and gets his ungrudged fee. Never mind, however, that very patient will some day return to you, will try to run down your neighbor, your so-called colleague, and you—well you will stop him from so doing.[5]

After the Russian pogroms of the 1880s, immigration to America increased dramatically, and the population exploded on the Lower East Side of New York. Many educated young men used the medical profession as a means of achieving upward social mobility (see chapter 16). In the 1890s the German Jewish medical elite condescended to serve their East Side brethren only in a consulting capacity. The newcomers were not acceptable to serve on the staff of Mount Sinai Hospital, and so in 1890 Beth Israel Hospital opened in a small house to accommodate the eastern European physicians. The physicians in the ghetto did their utmost to keep pace with the changing times, and several other hospitals were begun to serve the Hungarians, Austrians, and Russians, but all failed for lack of financial support.[6]

Jewish practitioners of that day knew that the best way to acquire a practice was to join as many lodges and societies as possible with the hope of being elected their doctor. The methods used to become a lodge doctor often were degrading, and the profession was discredited in the eyes of many. On the other hand, caring for Jewish patients was not easy and some accounts by physicians described a high degree of neurosis and anxiety among the East Siders:

> Tell an average Jew that his heart is "probably temporarily weak"—using any cautious if not scientific term—and during the next few months incessant inquiries will come in by all sorts of relatives and acquaintances of this patient, who will assail you with their own suggestions; you will learn that he has already been taken to a few specialists, that great sacrifices have been made

and that heaven and earth have been moved to take the man out of the office or shop, to treat him and overtreat him.[7]

In those days, medical examination was cursory at best—often no more than inspecting the tongue and checking the pulse. No matter, for the people believed that a good doctor could diagnose merely by looking at the patient. Many stories were told about physicians who never asked the patient what ailed him but prescribed only on the basis of what they saw. Patients didn't want to be examined either. What they expected and valued most were prescriptions; the more bitter and vile the more effectual they were considered. Doses before and after each meal, preferably silver- or gold-coated, were particularly impressive.

Of course, those were crude times. Given our modern sophistication, it is tempting to patronize, but it should be recalled that medical practice was unscientific until well into this century. Boston's physician-poet Dr. Oliver Wendell Holmes disparaged all of American medicine when he remarked in 1911 that "if the whole materia medica, as now used, could be sunk to the bottom of the sea, it would be all the better for mankind—and all the worse for the fishes."[8]

16

A G.P. Remembers

In 1965, Dr. Israel Augenblick was inspired to recount his memories of a half-century career as a general practitioner in New York City. A few selections from his unpublished 127-page manuscript are presented here, courtesy of the American Jewish Archives. The doctor's memoirs provide colorful descriptions of street and family life, but I will limit my selections to those that enlighten us about his choice of career and student experiences early in this century.[1]

Dr. Augenblick's background story is familiar. His father fled conscription into the Russian army by swimming across a river. In order to avoid identification, he changed the family surname from Augapfel to his wife's name, Augenblick. His mother was pregnant with him when they traveled to America in 1893. After a brief stay with an uncle in Newark, New Jersey, the Augenblicks settled on the Lower East Side. On the first floor of their three-story brownstone lived the family doctor, Dr. Gottesman, whom the young Augenblick admired because of his unpretentiousness, modesty, and concern for poor patients, to whom he listened with respect—"the attributes of the old time practicing physician."

Augenblick's parents would point out how the older sons of their friends were studying to become doctors, and he learned early that it was the greatest desire of the immigrant Jewish families to have a doctor son—only in this country could a child of poor parents achieve a place in such a noble profession. "I would listen to the conversation and was impressed by the repeated words 'My son, the doctor.'" When he attended the graduation of one of these young men, he was so inspired by the lofty speeches and recitation of the Hippocratic Oath, "I made up my mind that nothing could deter me from my ambition to become a physician."

Only a high school diploma or its equivalent was required in 1910, so at the age of sixteen Augenblick matriculated at Long Island College, situated in Brooklyn Heights. He recalled how during his third year, while observing a hysterectomy being performed by a famous obstetrician, Dr. John Polak, the doctor looked up in the middle of the operation, pointed at him, and said, "Doctor, will you come down and scrub up." He held abdominal retractors through the tense procedure and at the end was rewarded when Dr. Polak said, "Doctor, you will make a fine surgeon." Modestly, the student asked what he had done to earn such praise. "You assisted me very well. You haven't done anything to interfere with my work. Most of the assistants who help me are usually in my way when I'm operating. Thank you."

Dr. Augenblick described cases of lockjaw, diphtheria, caisson disease, gunshot wounds, and complicated obstetrical deliveries on kitchen tables. Most ex-

citing was ambulance duty at the Beekman Hospital—
careening horse-drawn wooden-wheeled vehicles, the
young doctor holding to straps to avoid being thrown.
Sometimes on the way back, he would ask the driver
to ride on Stanton Steet, where he lived, so that his
mother could see him. The driver would stop in front
of the house and press the pedal of the loud gong. Mrs.
Augenblick would look out of the window. "What un-
controllable emotion and joy she felt and how proud
she was seeing me dressed in a white duck uniform and
blue cap standing on the step in the rear of the ambulance. . . . What a thrilling and overwhelming delight I
experienced when I saw the smile on my mother's face.
A dream she waited for many years that finally came
true."

    After final written examinations, the final hurdles
to graduation were oral interviews with the senior faculty:

> I opened the door and walked in quietly. I could hear
> no sounds except the thumping and beating of my heart.
> In a low voice I said, "Good afternoon, gentlemen."
>   The professors and heads of the departments were
> seated in high leather upholstered chairs on the sides
> of a long mahogany table, at the head of which sat Dean
> Raymond. On the walls were portraits of the founders
> and prominent clinicians of the college. . . .
>   Dr. John A. McCorkle, professor of medicine, looked
> at me and in a husky voice asked, "Young man, what
> made you study medicine as a profession?"
>   I was always reticent and reserved in my speech, but
> at this time I answered quickly, "Living amongst the
> poor and watching the people struggle against depri-
> vation, hunger, and disease, I thought that I could do
> something as a doctor and humanitarian to alleviate
> their suffering and plight."

Professor Frank E. West then threw a question at me. "Doctor, what impressed you most during your attendance in college?"

I thought for a moment, then answered, "I believe that it was the way the professors taught the students, their sincerity in trying to make us good physicians."

At the conclusion of the conference Dean Raymond said, "Thank you. That is all."

He was sure that he had failed, and Augenblick and his classmates had to wait for weeks before they learned their fate. Then, the fateful day—"excitement, exhilaration and commotion prevailed. . . ."

Augenblick rode the subway home, wanting to call out his good fortune to strangers:

I entered my home, saw my mother and embraced her with tears flowing down my cheeks. "Mother," I said, crying. "It has happened. I am graduating. Your wish has come true after all these years. The day has finally arrived."

My mother cried and held my face between her hands, kissed me briefly on both cheeks, released them, then with a big hug said, "*Mein kind. Mein kind.* I knew that you would become a doctor. Thank God again for what he did for you and your parents."

The vignette wonderfully describes the special significance that a medical career held for immigrant Jewish families.

17

Women in
Medical Practice

Even in ancient times Jewish women may have engaged in medical practice. Indeed, many of the popular medical recipes of the Talmud are ascribed to Rabbi Abaye's foster mother or nursemaid, whose name has not been preserved.[1]

During the Middle Ages, there were sporadic mentions in official records of female Jewish physicians in Spain and Turkey. Sarah la Mirgesse practiced in Paris about 1292. In Marseille in 1326, Sara de Saint Gilles agreed to teach Salvet de Bourgneuf the art of medicine for a period of seven months as well as to board, lodge, and clothe him. None of these women attended medical school but acquired their knowledge mainly through reading books or through experience. Fifteen women practitioners, most of them Jewish, were known to be licensed in Frankfurt between 1387 and 1497, and Sara of Wurzberg was granted a license in 1419 and apparently had a lucrative practice and could afford to purchase an estate. In Poland, the municipal records of

Warsaw in 1435 cite a legal document concerning a
Jewish woman named Slava, the wife of a prominent
banker, who agreed to cure a certain Sushko for the sum
of 180 groshen—not a small amount in those days.[2, 3, 4]
During the Renaissance, women became relatively
emancipated and some were well educated and began
to engage in public life. Salerno in southern Italy, which
had emerged as one of the first medical centers, by the
tenth and eleventh centuries was famed for its skilled
female physicians, who were sometimes referred to as
"the women of Salerno." Italian female physicians did
not restrict their attentions to their own sex. A Jewess
named Virdimura was authorized to practice in Sicily
after examination in 1376 and stated that she wanted to
practice among the poor who were unable to pay the
large fees of other physicians.

The predominant obstetrical practitioners in rural
Russia until well into this century were village midwives.
During the Middle Ages, midwives were unskilled and
criticized by some as ignorant, dirty, and superstitious.[5]
Schools for midwives were opened in Paris at the end
of the sixteenth century, and gradually midwives began
to receive formal training. By the late eighteenth and
nineteenth centuries, a large percentage of Russian feldshers were women because of the establishment of
schools for midwives in 1757; subsequently these graduates were known as feldsher-midwifes.

The following account from a *shtetl* memorial book
describes such a feldsher-midwife:

> The real "crown" of the family was . . . Beila, the mid-
> wife of the "blessed hands." She was respected as the
> "mother" of the majority of the town's children. She was
> always busy and whenever attending a delivery, had

to prepare with her own hands all the necessary requirements; in many cases she had not been paid for her work at the birth of the previous child, but nevertheless would carry on quietly and efficiently. She continued to work until old age. . . . The respect the people had for Beila could be seen when she died and all the mothers lit candles at her deathbed and around her house. Thus, there were thousands of candles, a sight that no one would soon forget.[6]

Rachel Hirsch (1870–1953) was the first Jewish woman to receive the title of professor of medicine in Prussia (1913). She was the granddaughter of the founder of the neo-Orthodox movement in Germany, Samson Raphael Hirsch. Her pioneering research on renal physiology at Berlin's Charite Hospital was not taken seriously and was not "rediscovered" until fifty years later.

We tend to think of Jewish history only in terms of occidental or Middle Eastern experience, but an outstanding Jewish physician whose name is unknown in the West was Jerusha Jhirad (1891–1984), who was born into the Bene Israel community in Thane, a suburb of Bombay. There was no tradition of anti-Semitism in India, and Jhirad's major hurdle was to overcome prejudice against women who pursued professional careers. She was the first of her community to seek a medical career, and this was facilitated by her winning a scholarship to study in London. She obtained her medical degree in 1910 and then returned to Bombay, where she developed a flourishing practice in obstetrics-gynecology. Over her long career, Dr. Jhirad had many important responsibilities as a medical educator and administrator. In addition to her medical duties, she was a leader of the Indian Jewish community, and in 1925 she introduced "liberal Judaism" to the subcontinent. When she retired in 1947, she received many awards and signs of respect.[7]

Professional opportunities expanded for women in this century, and increasing numbers of Jewish women entered scientific careers and began to practice medicine so that today there is nothing unusual about their full participation. Two of three Jewish women who won Nobel Prizes in medicine and physiology were not physicians. The first was Gerty Theresa Radnitz Cori (1896–1957), who shared the award with her husband for their research in carbohydrate metabolism. Just thirty years later, Rosalyn Sussman Yalow was honored for her contributions in developing the radioimmunoassay, which permitted measurement of insulin and other hormones. She had collaborated for twenty-two years at the Bronx Veterans Administration Hospital with Dr. Solomon Berson.

Dr. Yalow was born in the Bronx of immigrant parents and was inspired to pursue a scientific career when she read the biography of Marie Curie. She overcame numerous hurdles and in her acceptance speech in Oslo in 1947 challenged young women to become scientists and use their talents to benefit all people. "We must believe in ourselves or no one else will believe in us."[8]

No account of Jewish medical practice would be complete without paying homage to the Jewish mother, ever formidable not only by virtue of her potent chicken soup and sometimes noxious home remedies but because of her single-mindedness in directing her sons to pursue careers in medicine or exhorting her daughters to marry doctors. As primary guardians of family health, Jewish mothers believed in the principle of preventive medicine; children should not get into a draft or get chilled and, above all, they should eat enough.

18

Racism and Jewish Health

The general state of Jewish health and medical practice has often had political implications. The following three examples from the eighteenth, nineteenth, and twentieth centuries are cited because they provide a social mirror of their times as they concerned the Jewish medical condition.

In the 1770s the Societe Royale de Medecine was charged by the French Crown with collecting information about the health of the general population. During this prerevolutionary period there was much idealistic debate about the rights of man and the proposition that all men are free and equal. The Jews, however, presented a problem. They didn't fit into the Christian world and were considered alien although they shared a common religious heritage. Some Jews, such as Moses Mendelssohn, advocated the end of communal separation, but if this were to be accomplished, the Jews would have to be integrated into the main society. Naysayers claimed that they suffered from disqualifying social and biological pathology.[1]

In 1781 a relatively obscure French physician named
Le Jau reported to the Societe on his experience in caring
for the small Ashkenazic population of Phalsbourg. The
Ashkenazim, unlike their more affluent and assimilated
Sephardic brethren, were seen as a group apart, imprisoned by custom, obsolete beliefs, and poverty. The following selected portions of Le Jau's report are instructive:

> Although the Jews live among the Christians, it is not
> difficult to perceive, if one only cares to see them close
> up, that they form a distinct nation in our towns and
> bourgs. This judgment will hardly appear curious to
> anyone who cares to examine how they exist, live, and
> conduct themselves among us. . . . Observation has
> given me proofs that there are some points of differ-
> ence in the diseases of Jews. . . . If observance of the
> law of Moses and of the Talmud benefits the Jews
> because of their frugality and their choice of meats and
> drink, their separation from other citizens contributes
> unfailingly to the gloom and melancholy that is seen
> among most of them. Indeed, how can their souls not
> be affected by their withdrawn and anxious lives and
> the humiliation to which they are reduced in spite of
> their wealth and money? . . . Jewish morals are unargu-
> ably better than those of the Christians; it is a rare thing
> for them to indulge in the debaucheries and excesses
> of our young people; but for all that they are no more
> robust. The reasons for this should be attributed to their
> tendency to melancholy and their early marriages. At a
> young age, an abundant loss of semen is a boundless
> source of weakness. To avoid "libertinage," fathers and
> mothers marry off their sons and especially their daugh-
> ters at an early age. As the Jews expect to find supreme
> happiness in the number of children they have, they
> engage in sex without restraint. These practices are
> responsible for the pallor and frailty commonly found
> in young couples.

Turning to Jewish culinary practice, Le Jau continued, "The food they eat is not without its faults; they often eat unleavened bread, and have a passion for cakes, pastries, and other delicacies. Such foods tend toward a corruption of the bodily fluids and a slackening of the fibers, and the most difficult part is when they permit their children and young people to take part in these domestic excesses, making them susceptible to diseases caused by crudity of the upper bowels, and by the viscosity and putridity of their humors."

Although today Le Jau's assessment seems unfair and harsh, he was not an anti-Semite. Indeed, similar observations were made by contemporary Jewish physicians such as Elcan Isaac Wolf, who in 1877 wrote a medical text in which he discussed the health characteristics of Mannheim's Jewish population. He suggested that Jewish worship depleted body and soul; for example, the use of ritual baths was debilitating in cold climates. Poor housing and sanitation in the crowded towns, improperly prepared food, anxiety to earn a living, and continual sorrow were thought to contribute to prevailing Jewish disorders, including hypochondriasis, melancholia, and hemorrhoids. Wolf believed that rural life was superior to urban life and advocated that Jews return to agriculture as during biblical times. He urged the use of simple foods rather than sharing one's money with the confectioner, the apothecary, and the doctor and warned against excess use of coffee and tea. He also railed against ignorant and quackish midwives, whom he said injured both mothers and infants and should be limited to their one useful purpose—giving enemas.

It should not be altogether surprising that one hundred years later, nearly the same descriptions were echoed in the United States. At the close of the nineteenth century the health status of immigrants was an issue that affected immigration policy, since it was feared that immigrants might infect others or that their poor health might make them unable to work and strain the economy.

In his book *Silent Travelers: Germs, Genes, and "The Immigrant Menace"*, Alan Kraut comments that for many of the newcomers,

> Better health as defined in American terms seemed to require relinquishing cherished customs, traditions, and trusted therapies on the altar of assimilation. . . . Overwhelmingly, members of the various ethnic groups turned to their own institutions, to their own physicians and care givers, especially in the early years after arrival, in an effort to obtain health care that did not require them to abandon their cultural identities. . . . Traditional healers and allopathic physicians of one hundred years ago often stood glaring at the bedside of a sick immigrant child, arguing that only his or her definition of the condition and therapy could save the patient.[2]

Jewish existence in nineteenth-century Russia was little different from medieval times, pitiful from the standpoint of health and sanitation. Yet in spite of their poverty, immigrant Jews often enjoyed better health than their neighbors. Kraut points out the irony that even as anti-Semitic critics portrayed the Jews as unclean, unhealthy, and disease-prone, statistics refuted these very notions. Data seemed to suggest that Jews were less susceptible to certain diseases than were their gentile neighbors, but this did not deter anti-Semites who were adept at distorting health statistics in order to prove that Jews and other groups were innately degenerate and a public health menace. In 1908 the medical director of the United States Navy complained, "The poorer classes of

Jews are unsanitary; they work and live in dirty and badly ventilated quarters. Though special virtue is claimed for the Jewish method of killing the animals they use for food, this is offset by the dirtiness of the shops in which the meat is sold."

As one racist observed, "On the physical side the Hebrews are the polar opposite of our pioneer breed. Not only are they undersized and weak muscled, but they shun bodily activity and are exceedingly sensitive to pain." An official government report published in 1890, *Vital Statistics of Jews in the United States*, was prepared in order to determine to what extent the Jews were assimilable and whether environmental conditions could level the playing field so that members of the "Jewish race" could find themselves able to achieve biological parity.

Among the Jewish physicians who attempted to refute racist arguments, Dr. Maurice Fishberg argued that of the homes of the poor in New York, the Jewish homes were the cleanest and the personal cleanliness of the Russian Jew was far above that of the average slum dweller. He insisted that their food was above reproach, that they had a cultural aversion to consumption of alcohol, and that they seemed to have a biological resistance to tuberculosis. Dr. Fishberg believed that the east European Jews' willingness to obtain medical attention from physicians and their habits of nutrition and hygiene accounted for their relatively low mortality rates and their resistance to particular diseases, such as syphilis, rather than innate racial characteristics.

Back in Europe, Jews frequently had been associated in the public mind with tuberculosis, which sometimes was regarded as "a Jewish disease" and was called "the tailor's disease" because so many consumptives were tailors. Again, this perception was refuted by the facts; statistics both in Europe and the United States indicated that mortality from TB was lower among the Jews than the gentiles. The explanation was uncertain. Some thought that the careful inspection of cattle for kosher certification reduced the potential for ingested infection. Others suggested that generations of close communal living led to a natural selection or adaptation process or that the rarity of alcoholism among Jews made them less predisposed. Socioeconomic factors certainly played a part, and the disease was more prevalent among the poor who lived in crowded urban enclaves. Regardless, it was clear that the children of the immigrants lived in better conditions and that life in America had a beneficial effect on the health of all its new citizens.

A different manifestation of medical anti-Semitism that has special resonance for our own time occurred in pre-World War II Germany. The German government had passed the first national health insurance plan in history as early as 1883. The system was run by "sickness funds" that were administered and paid for jointly by both employers and employees with the government playing a supervisory role. Much of the political debate anticipated current discussion in this country, but as the new system took hold it radicalized the medical profession. Physicians found themselves threatened by low wages and faced competition from other kinds of "doctors" or healers as well as from nonphysician managers.[3]

Jewish physicians played a disproportionate role in the worker health-care clinics, partly because of a commitment by Jewish physicians to public health and socialist programs, but also due to the fact that they settled in large urban centers where the clinics were most established. As a result, Jewish physicians were resented by their colleagues who wished to purge the sickness funds of Jews, socialists, or communists. Since Jews constituted about 14 percent of the medical profession and nearly 60 percent of panel doctors in Berlin, gentile physicians stood to benefit directly from their elimination. During the 1920s, as physicians' incomes fell both because of the weak economy and expansion of the national insurance system, they joined the Nazi Party in greater numbers than any other profession; from 1925 to 1944 the percentage of doctors in the party was almost three times as high as in the population as a whole.·

In the 1930s a series of new civil service regulations reduced Jewish physicians in the panels from nine thousand to about three thousand, and by the end of 1938 only 185 Jewish physicians still treated patients, six thousand had left the country or "disappeared," and about three thousand remained in Germany but were forbidden to practice. Among the results of the restructuring of the health system under the Third Reich was that Aryan physicians were rewarded by receiving monopoly powers so that nonphysician providers no longer could practice. In return, physicians found themselves carrying out the medical programs of the Reich.

19

Polish Hospitals and the Holocaust

During the Middle Ages, the first Jewish "hospitals" had been shelters for the poor and strangers and only occasionally for the sick. More accurately, they were hospices consisting of a single room or a little house near the Jewish cemetery or synagogue, referred to as a *hekdesh*, and the patients were cared for by the sick-care societies (*hevrah kaddisha*).[1]

In Poland, the first Jewish hospital was established in Cracow in the sixteenth century, and as time passed many similar hospitals were founded because of the insecurity of the Jewish population, their isolated life in the ghettos, and the persecution or actual banning of Jews from public institutions. Prior to the outbreak of World War II there were 48 Jewish hospitals in Poland, totaling 3,552 beds and representing 9 percent of all the hospitals in the country.

Space does not permit a detailed discussion of the catastrophic effects of the Nazi occupation on Jewish life in Europe, but since our focus has been on what the Jewish doctor's professional life was like during different historical periods, a single dismal example will be reported here as representative of this ghastly time.[2]

The city of Lodz had a Jewish hospital of 150 beds before World War II, but following the establishment of the ghetto it was closed and several factory lofts and other buildings in the ghetto were converted. Rudimentary equipment was donated by Jews and eventually more than 2,000 beds were opened. However, conditions were abysmal and thousands died of starvation and infectious diseases; tuberculosis, typhus, and typhoid were rampant.

A Jewish Department of Health was formed in October 1939, headed by Dr. Leon Szykier. Years later he recalled events of September 1942 in these words:

> The Germans threw the patients from the staircases, tore them from operating tables. . . . Everyone knew his destination—death. Some patients were saved thanks to the daring of the nurses and doctors. All this was accomplished by Dantesque scenes. Patients flung themselves from operating tables to evade the Germans. A woman with an abnormal pregnancy, on the operating table, ran off with an open abdomen and uterus. Twenty-four hours later she came back to complete the operation. Another one with a stomach operation jumped from the second floor and somehow succeeded in escaping. She is alive today. In the hospital on Mickiewicza Street, the patients escaped before the Germans surrounded the place. But all these efforts succeeded in rescuing only a small number of the patients. The bulk landed in the Chelmno death camp.

The following are diary notations of one of the survivors of the Lodz ghetto:

January 1941: Today Dr. Szykier returned from Warsaw.
He had gone there in the hope of bringing a few doctors . . . but none of them wanted to come to this
hellhole of Lodz.

April 18, 1941: Dr. Szykier called a meeting of the
doctors. Almost all of them came. They reported on the
dreadful ailments in the ghetto. There is no help. Many
sick people refuse treatment, seeking an early death.
In some rooms four to five patients lie in one bed and
one asks another: "When will death come?" At the end
of the meeting, Dr. Szykier gave information on the
number of visits by doctors in private dwellings. Between May 1940 and April 18, 1941, physicians visited
71,102 patients. The service has rendered aid to 94,355
persons. The Quick Help ambulance service was called
17,056 times. Some doctors work day and night. Six
doctors died recently because of overwork. Dr. Szykier
appealed to the doctors not to relax their efforts on
behalf of their people, who receive no aid from the
civilized world.

April 23, 1941: This week 100 Jews died. The first time
a few cases of spotted typhus have been registered.

June 20, 1941: An order from Berlin arrived today
stating that all mental cases are to be liquidated within
24 hours. There were 62 patients in the psychiatric
hospital. The Germans entered the hospital. One of the
murderers took out a list and began reading off names.
Those cited were loaded into a waiting car and the 62
were deported.

July 9, 1941: A terrible epidemic rages in the ghetto.
They call it dysentery. It claims hundreds of victims
daily. The doctors are helpless. They have no means
of curing it.

On May 12, the president of the *Judenrat* read a
letter from the Gestapo ordering all those suffering in-

curable diseases to be eliminated from the ghetto. On August 1, 1942, all hospitals were closed and some 2,000 patients were carted away to their death. Among them were 400 children and 80 pregnant women. Eighteen patients who attempted escape, but were caught, were shot to death. In three ghetto years Lodz Jewry lost 91,430 people.

After the war, an association of Jewish physicians from Poland called the Medical Alliance published a book that documented the story of their martyred colleagues and included brief biographies of more than twenty-five hundred physicians who perished during "the Hitler plague."

20

Academic Intolerance in America

Early in this century, many Jewish doctors became leaders in medical education and research, and their names could fill a "who's who" of the giants of modern medicine: Crohn, Dameshek, Friedberg, Janowitz, Libman, Master, Sabin, Salk, Waksman, Weinstein, Wintrobe, and thousands more. Early in their careers, many of these educators had to overcome professional and social prejudice at major universities. A consistent theme in their stories was how early in their careers opportunities were limited because of anti-Semitism in the basic sciences and in academic life. For this reason, most Jewish medical students gravitated to clinical fields where in hard times one could always make a living.

In the early 1900s, Jews sought to become physicians in far greater proportions than the youth of other segments of the society, until in 1920 medical school admissions committees began to impose quotas. Dr. Leon Sokoloff, who has studied this phenomenon, notes that in medicine the issue was not merely anti-Semitism but simple economics as a result of declining incomes during the Great Depression and then an influx of refugee physicians in the 1930s. To be sure, xenophobia permeated American society, particularly in the universities, but there were just too many medical schools and too many practitioners in the early days before academic standards were tightened.[1]

A national survey of Jewish physicians conducted by the Conference on Jewish Relations in 1936 indicated that most Jewish physicians practiced in the northeast. The study found that 47 percent (7,557) practiced in New York State, 9 percent in Illinois, 7 percent each in New Jersey and Pennsylvania, and 4 percent in California. The number of Jewish graduates of American medical schools increased dramatically at the beginning of the century in parallel with the waves of immigration: 277 graduated between 1896 and 1900; 460 from 1901 to 1905; 716 from 1906 to 1910; 977 from 1911 to 1915; and by 1931 to 1935 the number had grown to 2,313. Jewish physicians, when surveyed, indicated that they felt there were too many Jewish physicians; presumably they were concerned about competition from the influx of European immigrants. Nevertheless, most were doing well financially and had little difficulty getting hospital appointments. They also expressed concern about growing manifestations of anti-Semitism appearing within the United States at that time.[2]

In 1918, Columbia University devised a policy of "selective admissions" in order to limit enrollment of the burgeoning Jewish population of New York in favor of an elite "natural constituency." The result was a precipitous decline in Jewish enrollment. Graduates of New York's City College during the 1930s found it difficult to get into any medical school. Dr. Sokoloff quotes Nobel

Prize winner Dr. Arthur Kornberg, who was a City College graduate:

> In the grade schools and high schools of Brooklyn, I was enclosed in a circle of Jewish students and friends and was unaware of any anti-Semitism directed at me. This innocence persisted until my senior year at the academically prestigious City College of New York, whose student body was then 90 percent or more Jewish. Then came the disappointment of being rejected by virtually all of the many medical schools to which I applied. But it came as no surprise. I resented then that at the College of Physicians and Surgeons of Columbia University, a close neighbor of City College, an endowed scholarship for a City College graduate went begging for nine years because there were no candidates. To this day it rankles me.

In 1920, Yale University named Milton Charles Winternitz as dean of its medical school, one of the first Jews in the nation to hold a major position of academic leadership. Winternitz was a superb choice and during his tenure raised Yale from a second-rate institution to one of the finest in the world. As described by Dan A. Oren in his study of Jews at Yale, Winternitz was almost a caricature of the self-hating Jew striving to become part of gentile society. Brilliant, charismatic, inspirational, he also was abusive and terrifying to students and faculty alike. He was described as "a genius," "a bastard," "a leader," "a sadistic brute," and "one of the worst anti-Semites I ever met."[3]

Since Judaism was a badge of shame for Winternitz, he never would publicly admit that he was a Jew and worse, in order to achieve a "balanced" class, he introduced a quota system and instructed the admissions committee never to admit more than five Jews and two Italian Catholics and no blacks at all. Fifty percent to 60 percent of applicants for admission were "Hebrews," but he suggested that no more than 5 percent should be accepted, equal to the proportion of Jews in the general population. In the 1930s a 10 percent Jewish quota was common at many American medical schools, and the quota was much lower at some.

One positive result of the fierce competition caused by the quota systems was that only the most brilliant students succeeded and, no doubt, this natural selection process helps to account for the exemplary record of American Jewish physicians in recent decades. Many other students either sought careers in allied fields, such as dentistry or pharmacy, or went abroad for medical education to Scotland or Switzerland or Germany. More than 90 percent of Americans studying in European medical schools in 1932 and 1933 were Jewish.

By the 1950s, nearly 15 percent of American physicians were Jewish and the figure approached 50 percent for psychiatrists. In recent decades, however, the quota systems were gradually phased out so that today admissions practices are quite open. Nevertheless, efforts have been made to reimpose quotas in the name of affirmative action. For example, in the Bakke case of 1977, the United States Supreme Court stated that the University of California could not deny admission to a well-qualified white applicant in favor of a nonwhite candidate with lesser credentials solely on the basis of race.[4]

21

The Jewish Doctor in Literature

Many great novels have had medical protagonists, but generally, the novelist is most concerned with depicting the physician's personality within the context of the plot. Nevertheless, sometimes a vivid insight is provided into the profession itself. Consider the following remark about medical specialists that appears in Dostoyevsky's *The Brothers Karamazov*:

> I tell you, the old-fashioned doctor who treated all diseases has completely disappeared, now there are only specialists and they advertise all the time in the newspapers. If your nose hurts, they send you to Paris; there's a European specialist there, he treats noses. You go to Paris, he examines your nose: I can treat only your right nostril, he says. I don't treat left nostrils, it's not my specialty, but after me, go to Vienna, there's a separate specialist there who will finish treating your left nostril. What is one to do? I resorted to folk remedies.[1]

Of course, Dostoyevsky wasn't writing about Jewish doctors. The following descriptions enrich our understanding of Jewish physicians from the perspective of the novelist:

In *The Family Carnovsky* (1943), Israel Joshua Singer, the elder brother of Isaac Bashevis Singer, describes three generations of an Orthodox Polish family that during the late nineteenth century moves to Berlin, "the city of enlightenment." There, young George Carnovsky meets a busy and idealistic Jewish practitioner, Dr. Fritz Landau, who eventually becomes his medical role model. In truth, at first George is more smitten with the doctor's attractive daughter, herself a prospective medical student.[2]

Dr. Landau shows George an old medical book, saying, "You see, only a few hundred years ago, physicians treated the kings and princes with black magic potions and incantations. Now we have the X-ray machine and the microscope." The doctor has his patients completely undress for examination and exhorts them against smoking, drinking beer, or eating too much. "What do you expect from your stomach when you go on abusing it? You stuff it with meat, drown it with beer, and smother it with smoke so it growls, belches, fills with gas, and stinks like a garbage can." He talks bluntly to the women who he says pollute their bodies with grease, fat, sweets, coffee, and alcohol and then ask for medicines. He won't prescribe that "hogwash," that "colored water," for the way to health lies through adherence to the rules of hygiene. If in exceptional cases he does prescribe potions, pills, or powders, he makes them up in his own office. Needless to say, he draws the wrath of the pharmacists as well as his colleagues since he allows his patients to pay only as much as they can afford. If they need money, they are encouraged to take some from his collection tray.

In 1922, Sinclair Lewis, himself a Minnesota country doctor's son, listened to a heated debate about medical teaching and science and decided on the spot that would be the subject of his next novel. Among those present was a young bacteriologist, Paul Henry de Kruif, whom Lewis enlisted to serve as his scientific adviser. Out of their collaboration came Lewis's novel *Arrowsmith* as well as de Kruif's own classic *Microbe Hunters* (1926). De Kruif was responsible for the technical background of *Arrowsmith* and also was involved in the development of two major characters, the protagonist, Dr. Martin Arrowsmith, and his mentor, Professor Max Gottlieb.

In 1925, when Lewis was offered the Pulitizer Prize for *Arrowsmith* (he refused it), there was much speculation about who the prototypes for the characters were. Some suggested that Gottlieb was an amalgam of two of de Kruif's teachers, Professor F. G. Novy of the University of Michigan and Professor Jacques Loeb of Rockefeller Institute. Lewis later insisted that Gottlieb's personality was drawn from "as much as half a dozen other men" than Loeb, and it is plausible that among these may have been Paul Ehrlich, the Jewish immunologist who won the Nobel Prize in 1908. Ehrlich had discovered a treatment for syphilis—Salvarsan, popularly known as "606" or "the magic bullet"—and was one of de Kruif's heroes. In fact, his example inspired the impressionable young man to pursue a career in bacteriology. In *Microbe Hunters*, de Kruif writes, "So I love Paul Ehrlich . . . I love these microbe hunters. I love them for the men they are. I say they ARE for in my memory every man jack of them lives and will survive until this brain stops remembering."[3, 4, 5]

In the novel, Max Gottlieb was depicted as a world-famous immunologist, committed to long hours in the laboratory, aloof and scornful of commercialism in science. Born in Saxony in 1850, he had studied with Koch and Pasteur, married a gentile girl, achieved fame in research, and immigrated to America in 1890 in order to escape German militarism and anti-Semitism. He was described by his colleagues as "diabolist, pessimist, cynic, intellectual snob, pacifist, anarchist, atheist, Jew ...," more interested in pure science than in people.

He taught his students that "the ultimate lesson of science is to wait and doubt," sarcastically adding, "There are two kinds of M.D.'s—those to whom c.c. means cubic centimeter and those to whom it means compound cathartic. The second kind are more prosperous." At one point Lewis described the assimilated scientist in a reflective moment—"Gottlieb, the placidly virulent hater of religious rites, had a religious-seeming custom. Often, he knelt by his bed and let his mind run free. It was very much like prayer, though certainly there was no formal invocation, no consciousness of a Supreme Being—other than Max Gottlieb."

If Max Gottlieb was the kind of laboratory scientist who knew nothing about diagnosis or dosage, Dr. Samuel Adelman in Gerald Green's novel *The Last Angry Man* (1956) was a very different breed. Green's novel did not receive critical acclaim comparable to *Arrowsmith*, but it provided a picturesque description of the life of a physician at the lowest rung of professional success.[6]

Dr. Adelman, an immigrant from Rumania, was a general practitioner in a run-down Brooklyn neighborhood whose neighbors and patients were teenage hoodlums, kosher butchers, and policemen who rarely paid his small fees. This gruff, irascible man, who paradoxically loved gardening and reading Thoreau, was a fine clinician and a man of principle and integrity. He was unafraid to speak out or even to physically fight when he recognized an outrage of justice.

Green described a house call during the Spanish flu epidemic of 1918:

> The father is a barber and after paying the one dollar fee and walking him to the door asks, "Hey doc, okay if I use a cup?" "Cupping?" "Sure, cup, a match, you know. Bring up skin, bleed out bad blood." "You do and I'll punch your nose," the doctor said angrily. "What the hell you think this is, the Middle Ages? Don't you bleed that kid with cups or anything else." "No leech? Nice leech?" "No leeches, goddammit! She may get very sick before we're through. Grip they get better from. But she might get pneumonia, meningitis, an inflamed ear. So be careful. Listen to me for a change. Would I tell you how to cut hair?" . . . He knew that the barber would bleed his daughter anyway and while it would do no earthly good, it could not harm the little girl. For six years he had been warning patients not to employ cupping—*bankes* as his Jewish patients called it—knowing that they disobeyed his injunctions with impressive regularity.

Adelman's idol at Bellevue was Professor Harlow Brooks, who inquired what he planned to do after graduation.

"General practice." Brooks nodded. "The best kind. We'll have specialists for the right and left toe if we keep on. [Dostoyevsky would have agreed.] Medicine isn't drugs and surgery and therapy. Medicine is people. We deal in people, each one different, valuable, worthy of some kind of special attention. . . . Every year I live it seems to me there are less and less useful things to do in the world. Everything seems to be getting pallid, conformed, stereotyped, people as alike each other as one epithelial cell to another. Medicine is one of the few places where nothing is a waste, a drain, a bore. You can stay in one small village all your life, Adelman, and each day will present a new prospect, new things to learn, new gifts to impart to people. It's the difference between being a spectator and a participant. . . . You'll learn more and do more in one year of general practice in Brooklyn than in five years of postgraduate work."

What a splendid paean to primary-care practice captured in the expressive prose of the novelist! Common to the three fictitious physicians Landau, Gottlieb, and Adelman is that although none were religiously observant, in his own way each was an idealist who was passionately committed to serving either science or mankind. They were paragons of the secularized but fundamentally moral Jewish physician in conflict with a modern world that didn't share their values.

Conclusion

Having reviewed the lives of numerous court physicians, *shtetl rofim*, and world-famous scientists, can we now legitimately generalize about whether Jewish doctors have had any characteristics that distinguished them from their non-Jewish colleagues? It is tempting to be sentimental or self-serving, but except for their disproportionate numbers during various periods, it is difficult to convincingly answer the question in the affirmative. Jews may have excelled in medicine in some places and at some times, but they never were preeminent in all places and at all times, so one can't postulate a unique and enduring talent.

Comics might insist that the greatest Jewish contribution to medical therapy was chicken soup, but of course there was much more. Jewish scientists were pioneers in developing many of the most important pharmacologic advances—Ehrlich and Salvarsan, Salk and Sabin and the polio vaccine, Chain and penicillin, Waksman and streptomycin. Yet, one can question to what extent their Jewishness was instrumental in their genius.[1]

Medical historian Arturo Castiglioni summarized the evolution of Jewish medical thought as following a line from mystic and magic to empiric to scientific with an enduring feature being that ethical and hygienic concepts were accepted as having the authority of divine commands. No doubt this was true for many, and it is fair to suggest that even in modern times most Jewish physicians not only retained their intellectual vigor but also displayed the highest degree of professional integrity and served their communities with competence and devotion.[2]

For the most part, Jewish doctors were perceived as being intelligent, honest, and principled. Surely they must also have been competitive and courageous in order to succeed in the face of adversity. Many pursued the medical profession because therein lay an opportunity for social and economic improvement, and when they were allowed to enter the mainstream, they flourished on the basis of their own talents and diligence.

During times of trouble, no doubt, their first concern was personal survival, which was best accomplished by adapting to the circumstances. Only then could they focus on achieving professional success, and in this the traditional Jewish passion for knowledge and its abiding commitment to social justice were important attributes.

Is there any practical value in studying medical history? The pulmonologist Andre Cournand answered the question affirmatively in these words:

> In unfolding the common patrimony which unites successive generations of inquiring men, in meeting them

as individuals, in attempting to understand the problems they had to face, the intellectual climate in which
their investigations were pursued, and the historical
and social conditions under which they lived, it is my
belief that a sharper consciousness of our own nature
is brought forth. . . .[3]

Dr. Cournand's eloquent response applies equally
to Jewish and to general medical history, for when we
recall "our common patrimony," we celebrate and vali-
date it. Equally important, by so doing we achieve
heightened perspective and appreciation for our own
present endeavors.

Epilogue:
Bagels and *Bankes*

When I began writing this book, I was determined to have a catchy title and fancied "Bagels and *Bankes*." I confess that I loved the title, undignified as it was. It had alliteration and gastronomic appeal as well as a hint of mystery. Why not "Bagels and *Bankes*"? Because it was a gross misrepresentation. None of the essays in this collection discuss bagels and there is hardly any mention of the venerable medical technique of cupping, known as *bankes* (bahn-kuhs) in Yiddish. "Bagels and *Bankes*" was jettisoned with regret.

But perhaps I was too quick to submit to the advice of my sober critics who despised frivolity. After all, a cardiologist friend of mine eats a dry bagel every day for lunch. He suffers from heart disease and understands the importance of a low-fat diet. That is not to imply that bagels have unique medicinal value, but the fact is that throughout history physicians have admonished their patients to eat wisely. So have rabbis and Jewish mothers.

As for *bankes*, like bagels they were not exclusively a Jewish phenomenon. Cupping is an ancient remedy that dates back at least two millennia to the Egyptians and still is being used today, particularly in parts of Asia. It is based on ridding the body of whatever ails it and was used for a wide spectrum of complaints including pain, inflammation, poor appetite, headache, and cough. Cupping generally involved applying glass containers to the skin after first heating the inside with a burning candle. Depletion of oxygen created a vacuum so that the cup not only adhered to the skin but, in theory, sucked the deep-seated offending matter to the surface. The panacea was hardly "alternative medicine" since it was employed by such early medical giants as Hippocrates and Celsus and later by Sydenham, Heberden, Boerhaave, and Hunter.[1, 2]

Cupping was particularly prevalent in eastern Europe, and during New York City's great influenza epidemic in 1918, one observer commented that among the Russian Jewish immigrants it was "hard to find a living human being whose chest had not been cupped either as a prevention or as a cure for influenza or pneumonia." Many people were convinced of the efficacy of cupping, even if its physiologic effect was no more than that of a placebo or a counterirritant. Indeed, there was almost nothing for which it might not be beneficial except, as noted in a popular Yiddish definition of futility, "It will do him as much good as *bankes* for a corpse."

"Bagels and *Bankes*"? Alas!

Notes

INTRODUCTION

1. David B. Ruderman, *Jewish Thought and Scientific Discovery In Early Modern Europe* (New Haven and London: Yale University Press, 1995), pp. 286–287.

2. Harry Savitz, *Profiles of Erudite Jewish Physicians and Scholars* (Chicago: Spertus College of Judaica Press, 1973), p. 4.

3. Bernard Schlessinger and June Schlessinger, *The Who's Who of Nobel Prize Winners, 1901–1990* (Phoenix, AZ: Oryx Press, 1991).

4. Henry E. Sigerist, "The Social History of Medicine," *The Western Journal of Surgery, Obstetrics and Gynecology* 48 (1940): 715–722.

5. Thomas McKeown, "A Sociological Approach to the History of Medicine," *Medical History* 14 (1970): 342–351.

CHAPTER 1
AN HISTORICAL PERSPECTIVE

1. Fred Rosner, *Medicine in the Bible and the Talmud* (New York: Yeshiva University Press, 1977).

2. David Feldman, *Health and Medicine in the Jewish Tradition* (New York: Crossroad, 1986).

3. David Margalith, "Talmudic Maxims on Hygiene," *HaRofe HaIvri* 34 (1961): 208–210.

4. Julius Preuss, *Biblical and Talmudic Medicine*, ed. Fred Rosner (New York and London: Sanhedrin Press, 1978), pp. 11–33.

5. Stephen Newmyer, "Talmudic Medicine: A Classicist's Perspective," *Judaism* 29 (1980): 360–367.

6. Albert S. Lyons and R. Joseph Petrucelli II, *Medicine: An Illustrated History* (New York: Harry N. Abrams, 1978).

7. Henry E. Sigerist, *The Great Doctors* (New York: Doubleday Anchor Books, 1958), pp. 48–57.

8. Jonathan R. Hiatt and Nathan Hiatt, "Galen—A Father of Medicine," *Journal of the American College of Surgeons* 178 (1994): 410–416.

9. Hirsch J. Zimmels, *Magicians, Theologians and Doctors* (London: Edward Goldston & Son, 1952), p. 23.

10. E. Carmoly, *History of the Jewish Physicians*, trans. John Dunbar (Baltimore: John Murphy, 1845?), pp. 36–37.

11. Nancy G. Siraisi, *Medieval and Early Renaissance Medicine* (Chicago: University of Chicago Press, 1990), pp. 48–77.

12. Jane S. Gerber, *The Jews of Spain: A History of the Sephardic Experience* (New York: Macmillan, 1992), pp. 109–110.

13. Barbara W. Tuchman, *A Distant Mirror: The Calamitous 14th Century* (New York: Alfred A. Knopf, 1978), p. 109.

14. David B. Ruderman, *Science, Medicine, and Jewish Culture in Early Modern Europe* (Tel Aviv: Tel Aviv University, 1987), p. 9.

15. Howard Sachar, *Farewell Espana: The World of the Sephardim Remembered* (New York: Alfred A. Knopf, 1994), p. 33.

16. Edwin Mendelsohn, *The Pope's Jewish Doctors, 492–1655 c.e.* (Lauderhill, FL, 1991), p. 111.

17. Moses A. Shulvass, *The Jews in the World of the Renaissance* (Chicago: Spertus College of Judaica Press, 1973).

18. Cecil Roth, *The Jewish Contribution to Civilization* (Cincinnati, OH: The Union of American Hebrew Congregations, 1940), pp. 220–250.

19. Marquis de Custine, *Empire of the Czar: A Journey Through Eternal Russia (1839)* (New York: Anchor Books, 1989), p. 132.

20. Steven Beller, *Vienna and the Jews, 1867–1938: A Cultural History* (Cambridge: Cambridge University Press, 1989), pp. 33–43.

CHAPTER 2
EARLY JEWISH OPINIONS OF PHYSICIANS

1. Jane S. Gerber, *The Jews of Spain: A History of the Sephardic Experience* (New York: Macmillan, 1992), p. 16.

2. David S. Ruderman, *Science, Medicine and Jewish Culture in Early Modern Europe* (Tel Aviv: Tel Aviv University, 1987), p. 16.

3. Harry Friedenwald, *The Jews and Medicine*, vol. 1 (Baltimore: Johns Hopkins University Press, 1944), pp. 11–13.

4. Fred Rosner, "The Best of Physicians Is Destined for Gehenna," *New York State Journal of Medicine* 83 (1983): 970–972.

CHAPTER 3
MEDICAL OATHS AND APHORISMS

1. Hans-Georg Rupp, "The Oath of Asaph," *Koroth* 9 (1985): 205–210.

2. Fred Rosner and Sussman Muntner, "The Oath of Asaph," *Annals of Internal Medicine* 63 (1965): 317– 320.

3. Salo W. Baron, *A Social and Religious History of the Jews*, vol. 8, *Philosophy and Science* (Philadelphia: The Jewish Publication Society of America, 1958), p. 262.

4. Harry Friedenwald, *Jewish Luminaries in Medical History* (Baltimore: Johns Hopkins University Press, 1946), pp. 6–7.

5. Harry Friedenwald, *The Jews and Medicine*, vol. 1 (Baltimore: Johns Hopkins University Press, 1944), pp. 24–26.

6. Friedenwald, *Jewish Luminaries*, p. 16.

7. Friedenwald, *Jews and Medicine*, pp. 273–279.

8. Harry Savitz, *Profiles of Erudite Jewish Physicians and Scholars* (Chicago: Spertus College of Judaica Press, 1973), p. 13.

CHAPTER 4
MAIMONIDES, "THE EAGLE OF PHYSICIANS"

1. David Druck, *Yehuda Halevi, His Life and Works* (New York: Bloch Publishing Company, 1941), p. 48.

2. Fred Rosner, "Moses Maimonides (1135 to 1204),"
Annals of Internal Medicine 62 (1965): 372–375.

3. Fred Rosner, *Maimonides' Medical Writings* (Haifa:
The Maimonides Research Institute, 1984).

4. Abraham Joshua Heschel, *Maimonides: A Biography* (New York: Farrar, Strauss and Giroux, 1982),
pp. 214–215.

5. Fred Rosner, *Medicine in the Mishneh Torah of
Maimonides* (New York: Ktav, 1984), pp. 82–84.

6. Salo W. Baron, *A Social and Religious History of
the Jews*, vol. 8, *Philosophy and Science* (Philadelphia:
The Jewish Publication Society of America, 1958), p. 251.

7. Harry Friedenwald, *Jews and Medicine*, vol. 1
(Baltimore: Johns Hopkins Press, 1944), pp. 198–199.

8. Jacob Minkin, *The World of Moses Maimonides*
(New York and London: Thomas Yoseloff, 1957), pp. 149–
151.

CHAPTER 5
THE PERILS OF COURT LIFE

1. W. M. Feldman, "Jewish Contributors to Medical Knowledge," *The Jewish Forum* 14 (1931): 234.

2. Will Durant, *The Renaissance: A History of Civilization in Italy from 1304–1567 A.D.* (New York: Simon
and Schuster, 1953), p. 531.

3. W. H. Gantt, *Russian Medicine* (New York: Hoeber,
1931), pp. 24–25.

4. Cecil Roth, *The Jews in the Renaissance* (Philadelphia: The Jewish Publication Society of America,
1959), pp. 216–220.

5. Noah Shapiro, "The Belief in the Curative Powers of Precious Stones Among the Jews," *HaRofe HaIvri*
25 (1952): 158–160.

6. Harry Friedenwald, *Jews and Medicine*, vol. 2 (Baltimore: Johns Hopkins Press, 1944), pp. 468–496.

7. Edward Kossoy and Abraham Ohry, *The Feldshers* (Jerusalem: The Magnes Press, 1992), pp. 158–159.

8. Friedenwald, *Jews and Medicine*, pp. 757–758.

9. Ibid., pp. 736–737.

CHAPTER 6
BLACK BILE AND BLACK DEATH
IN RENAISSANCE ITALY

1. Luis Garcia-Ballester, "Dietetic and Pharmacological Therapy: A Dilemma Among 14th Century Jewish Practitioners in the Montpellier Area," *Clio Medica* 22 (1991): 23–37.

2. Harry Friedenwald, *Jews and Medicine*, vol. 1 (Baltimore: Johns Hopkins University Press, 1944), pp. 332–403.

3. Arthur Teller, *The Wellspring of Living Waters by Issachar Bar Teller, Physician and Surgeon* (New York: Tal Or Oth, 1988), p. 103 n. 156.

4. David Ruderman, *Kabbalah, Magic, and Science: The Cultural Universe of a Sixteenth-Century Jewish Physician* (Cambridge: Harvard University Press, 1988), pp. 32–44.

CHAPTER 7
PADUA'S UNIQUE INFLUENCE

1. Jerome J. Bylebyl, "The School of Padua: Humanistic Medicine in the 16th century," in *Health, Medicine and Mortality in the 16th Century*, ed. Charles Webster (Cambridge: Cambridge University Press, 1979), pp. 335–370.

2. Jacob Shatzky, "On Jewish Medical Students of Padua," *Journal of the History of Medicine* 5 (1950): 444–447.

3. David B. Ruderman, "Science, Medicine and Jewish Culture in Early Modern Europe," in *Spiegel Lectures in Early Jewish History,* #7 (Tel Aviv: Tel Aviv University, 1987), pp. 5–25.

4. D. A. Friedman, "Joseph Shelomoh Delmedigo," *Medical Leaves* 4 (1942): 83–94.

5. Jacob R. Marcus, *Communal Sick-Care in the German Ghetto* (Cincinnati: Hebrew Union College Press, 1947), pp. 27–30.

6. Nigel Allan, "A Jewish Physician in the Seventeenth Century," *Medical History* 28 (1984): 324–328.

7. Leon Wulman, "History of Jewish Physicians and Medical Institutions," in *The Martyrdom of Jewish Physicians in Poland,* ed. Louis Falstein (New York: Exposition Press, 1963), pp. 19–20.

8. Hirsch J. Zimmels, *Magicians, Theologians and Doctors* (London: Edward Goldston & Son, 1952), pp. 98, 144.

9. David B. Ruderman, *Jewish Thought and Scientific Discovery in Early Modern Europe* (New Haven and London: Yale University Press, 1995), p. 111.

10. Wulman, "History of Jewish Physicians," p. 34.

11. Ruderman, "Science, Medicine and Jewish Culture," pp. 23–25.

CHAPTER 8
DEFENSIVE MEDICINE

1. Harry Friedenwald, *Jewish Medical Luminaries* (Baltimore: Johns Hopkins University Press, 1946), p. 18.

2. Harry Friedenwald, *Jews and Medicine*, vol. 2 (Baltimore: Johns Hopkins University Press, pp. 448–452.

CHAPTER 9
PORTUGUESE MIGRANTS.

1. Harry Friedenwald, *Jews and Medicine*, vol. 1 (Baltimore: Johns Hopkins University Press, 1944), pp. 307–321.

2. Ivan A D'Cruz, "Garcia da Orta in Goa: Pioneering Tropical Medicine," *British Medical Journal* 303 (1991): 1593–1594.

3. Fred Rosner, "Jewish Contributions to Medicine in the United States: 1776–1976," *New York State Journal of Medicine* 76 (1976):1327–1332.

4. Robert Shosteck, "Dr. John de Sequeyra—Early Virginia Physician," *American Jewish Archives* 23 (1971): 198–212.

5. Thomas J. Tobias, "The Many-Sided Dr. La Motta," *American Jewish Historical Quarterly* 50 (1961): 200–218.

6. Desmond G. Julian, "Jacob Mendez Da Costa," *Journal of Medical Biography* 1 (1993): 248–252.

CHAPTER 10
EIGHTEENTH-CENTURY MEDICAL VIGNETTES

1. Hirsch J. Zimmels, *Magicians, Theologians and Doctors* (London: Edward Goldston & Son, 1952), pp. 37–140.

2. Solomon Maimon, *An Autobiography* (Boston: Cupples & Hurd, 1888), pp. 94–95.

3. Leon Wulman, "History of Jewish Physicians and

Medical Institutions," in *The Martyrdom of Jewish Physicians in Poland*, ed. Louis Falstein (New York: Exposition Press, 1963), pp. 33–34.

4. Ibid., p. 32.

5. Harry Savitz, *A Jewish Physician's Harvest* (New York: Ktav, 1979), pp. 15–16.

6. Margaret Pelling and Charles Webster, "Medical Practitioners," in *Health, Medicine and Mortality in the Sixteenth Century*, ed. Charles Webster (Cambridge: Cambridge University Press, 1979), p. 185.

7. Alex Sakula, "The Doctors Schomberg and the Royal College of Physicians: An Eighteenth-Century Shemozzle," *Journal of Medical Biography* 2 (1994): 113–119.

CHAPTER 11
WHO REALLY WROTE "MAIMONIDES' PRAYER"?

1. Emil Bogen, "The Daily Prayer of a Physician," *Journal of the American Medical Association* 92 (1929): 2128.

2. Brigitte Ibing, "Markus Herz, a Biographical Study," *Koroth* 9 (1985): 113–121.

3. Raphael Patai, *The Jewish Mind* (New York: Charles Scribner's Sons, 1977), p. 248.

CHAPTER 12
THE LATE ENTRY OF RUSSIAN PHYSICIANS

1. Raphael Patai, *The Jewish Mind* (New York: Charles Scribner's Sons, 1977), pp. 216–217.

2. David Margalith, "Wonderworkers and Folk Healers," *HaRofe HaIvri* 34 (1961): 211–215.

3. Hirsch J. Zimmels, *Magicians, Theologians and Doctors* (London: Edward Goldston & Son, 1952), p. 20.

4. Ibid., pp. 22–23.

5. Noah Shapira, "Baruch Schick of Shklov," *HaRofe HaIvri* 35 (1962): 193–196.

6. Raphael Mahler, *A History of Modern Jewry, 1780–1815* (New York: Schocken, 1971), pp. 570–572.

7. Leon Wulman, "History of Jewish Physicians and Medical Institutions," in *The Martyrdom of Jewish Physicians in Poland*, ed. Louis Falstein (New York: Exposition Press, 1963), p. 38.

8. *Encyclopaedia Judaica* 4: 671.

9. Edward Kossoy and Abraham Ohry, *The Feldshers* (Jerusalem: The Magnes Press, 1982), p. 159.

10. Jacob S. Raisin, *The Haskalah Movement in Russia* (Philadelphia: The Jewish Publication Society of America, 1913), pp. 240–241.

11. Nancy M. Frieden, *Russian Physicians in an Age of Reform and Revolution, 1856–1905* (Princeton: Princeton University Press, 1981), pp. 22–26.

12. Harry Savitz, *Profiles of Erudite Jewish Physicians and Scholars* (Chicago: Spertus College of Judaica Press, 1973), pp. 56–61.

13. Ibid., pp. 53–55.

14. Arnold Margolin, *The Jews of Eastern Europe* (New York: T. Seltzer, 1926), pp. 95–108.

15. Meir Yoeli, "Shaul Tchernichovsky," *New England Journal of Medicine* 272 (1965): 1173.

CHAPTER 13
"MY SON THE FELDSHER"

1. Edward Kossoy and Abraham Ohry, *The Feldshers* (Jerusalem: The Magnes Press, 1992), pp. 27–33.

2. Arthur Teller, *The Wellspring of Living Waters by Issachar bar Teller, Physician and Surgeon* (New York: Tal Or Oth, 1988), pp. 1–8.

3. Samuel Ramer, "Who was the Russian Feldsher?" *Bulletin of the History of Medicine* 50 (1976): 213–225.

4. Victor W. Sidel, "Feldshers and 'Feldsherism,'" *New England Journal of Medicine* 278 (1968): 934–938, 987–992.

5. A. A. Roback, "Physicians in Jewish Folklore," *Medical Leaves* 4 (1942): 113.

CHAPTER 14
SHTETL MEDICINE

1. Chaim Aronson, *A Jewish Life Under the Tsars* (Totowa, NJ: Allanheld, Osmun, 1983), p. 13.

2. K. Bilgoray, "The Healer in Bilgoray," in *From a Ruined Garden*, ed. J. Kugelmass and J. Boyarin (New York: Schocken, 1983), p. 95.

3. Mark Zborowski and Elizabeth Herzog, *Life Is With People* (New York: International Universities Press, 1952), p. 355.

4. Harry Friedenwald, "The Evil Eye (*Ayin Haraah*)," *Medical Leaves* 3 (1939): pp. 44–47.

5. Shlomo Riskin, "Seeing God Means Being Blind to the Evil Eye," *The Jewish Week*, 17–23 December 1993, 57.

6. Joshua Trachtenberg, *Jewish Magic and Superstition: A Study in Folk Religion* (Philadelphia: The Jewish Publication Society of America, 1961).

7. Abraham Blinderman, "Isaac Bashevis Singer, Medicinal Fiction," *New York State Journal of Medicine* 81 (1981): 1382–1391.

CHAPTER 15
THE LOWER EAST SIDE

1. Joseph Hirsch and Beka Doherty, *The First Hundred Years of The Mount Sinai Hospital of New York, 1852–1952* (New York: Random House, 1952), pp. 1–13.

2. Solomon R. Kagan, *Jewish Contributions to Medicine in America* (Boston: Boston Medical Publishing Company, 1934), pp. 140–143.

3. Isaac A. Abt, "Abraham Jacobi," *Medical Leaves* 6 (1937): 11–13.

4. M. A. Lipkind, "Some East Side Physicians at the Close of the 19th Century," *Medical Leaves* 9 (1940): 106.

5. Abraham Jacobi, "The Modern Doctor," *New York Medical Journal and Philadelphia Medical Journal,* 24 June 1905, 1270.

6. A. J. Rongy, "Unusual Consultations," *Medical Leaves* 9 (1940): 120.

7. B. Liber, "The Behavior of the Jewish and Non-Jewish Patient: A Comparison," *Medical Leaves* 9 (1940): 159.

8. Robert L. Martensen, "Oliver Wendell Holmes, M.D.: An Appreciation," *Journal of the American Medical Association* 272 (1994): 1249.

CHAPTER 16
A G.P. REMEMBERS

1. Israel Augenblick, "I Remember: Nostalgic Memories of Half a Century in New York," unpublished manuscript housed at the American Jewish Archives, Cincinnati, OH, 1965.

CHAPTER 17
WOMEN IN MEDICAL PRACTICE

1. Julius Preuss, *Biblical and Talmudic Medicine*, ed. Fred Rosner (New York and London: Sanhedrin Press, 1978), p. 21.

2. Nancy G. Siraisi, *Medieval and Early Renaissance Medicine* (Chicago: University of Chicago Press, 1990), pp. 27–31.

3. Cecil Roth, *The Jews in the Renaissance* (New York: Harper Torchbooks, 1959), p. 50.

4. Leon Wulman, "History of Jewish Physicians and Medical Institutions," in *The Martyrdom of Jewish Physicians in Poland*, ed. Louis Falstein (New York: Exposition Press, 1963), p. 4.

5. Hirsch J. Zimmels, *Magicians, Theologians and Doctors* (London: Edward Goldston & Son, 1952), p. 32.

6. Edward Kossoy and Abraham Ohry, *The Feldshers* (Jerusalem: The Magnes Press, 1992), p. 162.

7. A. Jhirad, *A Dream Realized: Biography of Dr. Jerusha J. Jhirad* (Bombay: ORT Publications, 1990).

8. *Current Biography Yearbook*, ed. Charles Moritz (New York: H. W. Wilson Company, 1978), p. 113.

CHAPTER 18
RACISM AND JEWISH HEALTH

1. Harvey Mitchell and Samuel S. Kotteck, "An Eighteenth Century Medical View of the Diseases of the Jews in Northeastern France: Medical Anthropology and the Politics of Jewish Emancipation," *Bulletin of the History of Medicine* 67 (1993): 248–281.

2. Alan M. Kraut, *Silent Travelers: Germs, Genes and*

the "Immigrant Menace" (New York: Basic Books, 1994), p. 141.

3. Donald W. Light, Stephan Liebfried, and Florian Tennstedt, "Social Medicine vs. Professional Dominance: The German Experience," *American Journal of Public Health* 76 (1986): 78–83.

CHAPTER 19
POLISH HOSPITALS AND THE HOLOCAUST

1. Samuel S. Kottek, "The Hospital in Jewish History," *Reviews of Infectious Diseases* 3 (1981): 636–639.

2. Joseph Tenenbaum, "Jewish Medical Life Under Nazi Rule," in *The Martyrdom of Jewish Physicians in Poland*, ed. Louis Falstein (New York: Exposition Press, 1963), pp. 208–211.

CHAPTER 20
ACADEMIC INTOLERANCE

1. Leon Sokoloff, "The Rise and Decline of the Jewish Quota in Medical School Admissions," *Bulletin of the New York Academy of Medicine* 68 (1992): 497–517.

2. Jacob Goldberg, "Jews in Medicine: A National Survey," *HaRofe HaIvri* 10 (1936): 157–167.

3. Dan A. Oren, *Joining the Club: A History of Jews and Yale* (New Haven: Yale University Press, 1985), pp. 139–155.

4. G. H. Brieger, "Getting Into Medical School in the Good Old Days: Good for Whom?" *Annals of Internal Medicine* 119 (1993): 1138–1148.

CHAPTER 21
THE JEWISH DOCTOR IN LITERATURE

1. Fyodor Dostoyevsky, *The Brothers Karamazov* (Chicago: Encyclopaedia Britannica Inc., 1952), p. 340.

2. Israel Joshua Singer, *The Family Carnovsky* (New York: Vanguard Press, 1943), p. 93.

3. Sinclair Lewis, *Arrowsmith* (Cutchogue, NY: Bucaneer Books, Inc., 1976).

4. Paul de Kruif, *Microbe Hunters* (New York: Harcourt, Brace and World, 1926).

5. M. Schorer, *An American Life* (New York: McGraw Hill, 1961), pp. 367–419.

6. Gerald Green, *The Last Angry Man* (New York: Charles Scribner's Sons, 1956).

CONCLUSION

1. David L. Cowen, "The History of Pharmacy and History of the Jews," in *Feltschrift fur A. Lutz und J. Buchi* (Zurich: Juris Druck, 1983), p. 81.

2. Arturo Castiglioni, "The Contribution of the Jews to Medicine," in *The Jews: Their History, Culture and Religion*, ed. Louis Finkelstein (New York: Harper & Brothers, 1936), pp. 1349–1375.

3. Andre F. Cournand, *Circulation of the Blood*, ed. A. P. Fishman and D. W. Richards, pt. 1, chap. 1, quoted in *Familiar Medical Quotations*, ed. Maurice Strauss (Boston: Little, Brown and Company, 1968), p. 215.

EPILOGUE:
BAGELS AND *BANKES*

1. Constantine Kouskoukis, "Cupping: The Art and Value," *The American Journal of Dermatopathology* 5 (1983): 235–239.

2. J. L. Turk and Elizabeth Allen, "Bleeding and Cupping," *Annals of the Royal College of Surgeons of England* 65 (1983): 128–131.

Select Bibliography

Baron, Salo W. *A Social and Religious History of the Jews.* Vol. 8. Philadelphia: The Jewish Publication Society of America, 1958.

Beller, Steven. *Vienna and the Jews, 1867–1938: A Cultural History.* Cambridge: Cambridge University Press, 1989.

Falstein, Louis, ed. *The Martyrdom of Jewish Physicians in Poland.* New York: Exposition Press, 1963.

Feldman, David. *Health and Medicine in the Jewish Tradition.* New York: Crossroad, 1986.

Finkelstein, Louis, ed. *The Jews: Their History, Culture and Religion.* New York: Harper and Brothers, 1936.

Frieden, Nancy M. *Russian Physicians in an Age of Reform and Revolution, 1856–1905.* Princeton, NJ: Princeton University Press, 1981.

Friedenwald, Harry. *The Jews and Medicine,* 2 vols. Baltimore: Johns Hopkins University Press, 1944.

———. *Jewish Luminaries in Medical History.* Baltimore: Johns Hopkins University Press, 1946.

Gantt, W. H. *Russian Medicine*. New York: Hoeber, 1931.

Gerber, Jane S. *The Jews of Spain: A History of the Sephardic Experience*. New York: Macmillan, 1992.

Hirsch, Joseph, and Doherty, Beka. *The First Hundred Years of the Mount Sinai Hospital of New York, 1852–1952*. New York: Random House, 1952.

Kagan, Solomon R. *Jewish Contributions to Medicine in America*. Boston: Boston Medical Publishing Company, 1934.

————. *Jewish Medicine*. Boston: Medical-History Press, 1952.

Kossoy, Edward, and Ohry, Abraham. *The Feldshers*. Jerusalem: The Magnes Press, 1992.

Kraut, Alan M. *Silent Travelers: Germs, Genes and the "Immigrant Menace."* New York: Basic Books, 1994.

Lyons, Albert S., and Petrucelli, Joseph R. *Medicine: An Illustrated History*. New York: Harry N. Abrams, 1978.

Mahler, Raphael. *A History of Modern Jewry, 1780–1815*. New York: Schocken, 1971.

Margolin, Arnold. *The Jews of Eastern Europe*. New York: T. Seltzer, 1926.

Minkin, Jacob. *The World of Moses Maimonides*. New York and London: Thomas Yoseloff, 1957.

Oren, Dan A. *Joining the Club: A History of Jews and Yale*. New Haven: Yale University Press, 1985.

Patai, Raphael. *The Jewish Mind*. New York: Charles Scribner's Sons, 1977.

Preuss, Julius. *Biblical and Talmudic Medicine*, ed. Fred Rosner. New York and London: Sanhedrin Press, 1978.

Raisin, Jacob S. *The Haskalah Movement in Russia*. Philadelphia: The Jewish Publication Society of America, 1913.

Ravitch, Michael. *The Romance of Russian Medicine.* New York: Liveright Publishing Corp., 1937.

Rosner, Fred. *Medicine in the Bible and the Talmud.* New York: Yeshiva University Press, 1977.

————. *Medicine in the Mishneh Torah of Maimonides.* New York: Ktav, 1984.

————. *Maimonides' Medical Writings.* Haifa: The Maimonides Research Institute, 1984.

Roth, Cecil. *The Jewish Contribution to Civilization.* Cincinnati, OH: The Union of American Hebrew Congregations, 1940.

Roth, Cecil. *The Jews in the Renaissance.* Philadelphia: The Jewish Publication Society of America, 1959.

Ruderman, David. *Jewish Thought and Scientific Discovery in Early Modern Europe.* New Haven and London: Yale University Press, 1995.

Ruderman, David. *Kabbalah, Magic and Science: The Cultural Universe of a Sixteenth-Century Jewish Physician.* Cambridge: Harvard University Press, 1988.

Sachar, Howard. *Farewell Espana: The World of the Sephardim Remembered.* New York: Alfred A. Knopf, 1994.

Savitz, Harry. *A Jewish Physician's Harvest.* New York: Ktav, 1979.

Savitz, Harry. *Profiles of Erudite Jewish Physicians and Scholars.* Chicago: Spertus College of Judaica Press, 1973.

Shulvass, Moses A. *The Jews in the World of the Renaissance.* Chicago: Spertus College of Judaica Press, 1973.

Sigerist, Henry E. *The Great Doctors.* New York: Doubleday Anchor Books, 1958.

Siraisi, Nancy. *Medieval and Early Renaissance Medicine.* Chicago: University of Chicago Press, 1990.

Trachtenberg, Joshua. *Jewish Magic and Superstition: A Study in Folk Religion*. Philadelphia: The Jewish Publication Society of America, 1961.

Webster, Charles. *Health, Medicine and Mortality in the 16th Century*. Cambridge: Cambridge University Press, 1979.

Zborowski, Mark, and Herzog, Elizabeth. *Life Is With People*. New York: International Universities Press, 1952.

Zimmels, Hirsch J. *Magicians, Theologians and Doctors*. London: Edward Goldston & Son, 1952.

Index

151

About the Author

Michael A. Nevins, M.D., has practiced internal medicine and cardiology in northern New Jersey since 1968. He grew up in the Bronx, New York, and graduated from Dartmouth College and Tufts University School of Medicine. A former governor of New Jersey's chapter of the American College of Physicians, he was awarded that organization's Laureate Award in 1991 for career contributions in bioethics, geriatrics, and medical education. Dr. Nevins has published more than 70 articles in medical journals and is the author of *Dubrowa: Memorial to a Shtetl* (1982). Dr. Nevins and his wife, Phyllis, live in River Vale, New Jersey, and have three grown children, Andrea (Sherman), Daniel, and Ted.